CSIRO LOW-CARB EVERY DAY

BY PROFESSOR GRANT BRINKWORTH
AND PENNIE TAYLOR

Photography by
Jeremy Simons

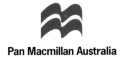
Pan Macmillan Australia

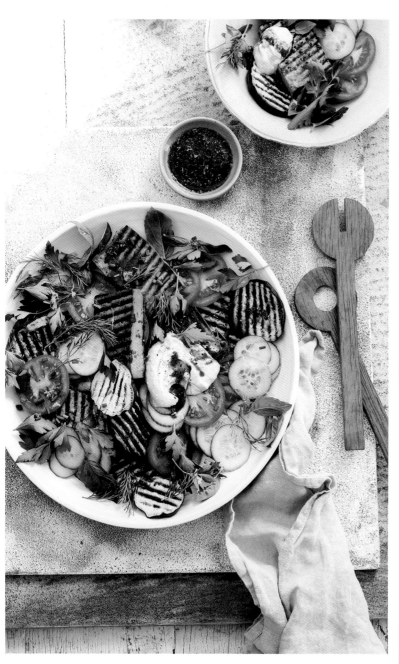
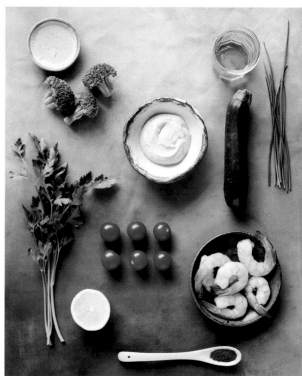
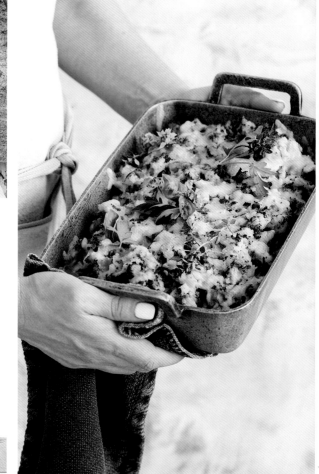
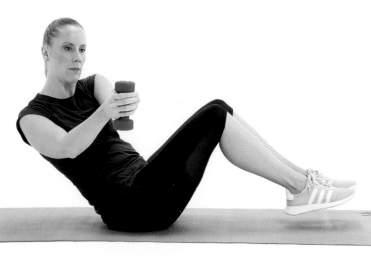

CONTENTS

AUTHOR AND CONTRIBUTOR PROFILES

Authors

Professor Grant Brinkworth

Grant is a principal research scientist in Clinical Nutrition and Exercise at CSIRO Health and Biosecurity. He has a PhD and expertise in diet, nutrition and exercise science. He has more than 17 years' experience leading large-scale, multidisciplinary clinical research teams and studies evaluating the effects of dietary patterns, foods, nutritional components and physical exercise on weight loss, metabolic disease risk management, health and performance.

Grant has particular interests in developing effective lifestyle solutions for achieving optimal weight, metabolic health and diabetes management, and understanding the role of lower-carbohydrate dietary patterns for health management. He has published more than 75 peer-reviewed research papers on the topic of diet and lifestyle management of obesity and related diseases. Grant is a recipient of a CSIRO medal and distinguished awards for research excellence and is an Adjunct Research Professor at the University of South Australia. He also holds an MBA degree, and has interests in innovation and the commercialisation of science outcomes and lifestyle programs for large-scale uptake and community adoption.

Pennie Taylor

Pennie is a senior research dietitian at CSIRO Health and Biosecurity. She is a contributor to the CSIRO range of programs, which aim to maximise health and wellbeing through better nutrition, physical activity and weight management.

Her expertise focuses on the development and delivery of novel dietary patterns, food and meal development, and commercialisation of health programs that aim to improve the health of the overweight and diabetic population. She has managed and supported many clinical trials exploring the influence of dietary patterns on health outcomes. Pennie is also a private practitioner for EvolvME and an active committee member for the Dietitians Association of Australia. For her PhD she investigated novel strategies to optimise glucose control, appetite responses and feeding behaviour in people with type 2 diabetes.

Contributors

Dr Natalie Luscombe-Marsh Natalie is a research scientist at CSIRO Health and Biosecurity, and an Adjunct Senior Lecturer at the University of Adelaide. She has a PhD in nutrition and disease, and more than 12 years' experience in designing clinical trials determining the acute and longer-term effects of different dietary patterns, particularly those higher in protein and unsaturated fat, on cardiometabolic risk in obesity and type 2 diabetes. A major focus of her research has been understanding the role gut mechanisms play in the regulation of energy intake and glycaemia in response to protein, in young and older adults. Natalie has authored 50 peer-reviewed papers, two book chapters, and numerous industry reports, and has received several awards recognising the novelty and impact of her work.

Dr Tom Wycherley Tom is a lecturer and research scientist at the University of South Australia. He is an accredited exercise scientist and holds a PhD in nutrition and exercise science, and a master's degree in epidemiology. He has more than 10 years' experience researching the role of dietary intake and physical activity in regulating body weight and cardiometabolic disease risk. He has published more than 30 peer-reviewed research articles, and is passionate about translating research findings into improved public health.

Professor Campbell Thompson Campbell is a senior consultant in medicine at the Flinders Medical Centre and the Royal Adelaide Hospital. He has spent more than 10 years on metabolic research using magnetic resonance and other biochemical techniques to monitor high-energy and fat metabolism at rest and during exercise in adults, elite athletes and children. He has a particular interest in metabolic syndrome, insulin resistance and diabetes. Since 2009, Campbell has worked in the Comprehensive Metabolic Care Centre at the Royal Adelaide Hospital, where weight-management strategies such as bariatric (weight-loss) surgery are offered to overweight people. He has written more than 150 peer-reviewed research articles.

Professor Manny Noakes Manny is the Research Director for the Nutrition and Health Program at the CSIRO. She was instrumental in the development and release of five editions of *The CSIRO Total Wellbeing Diet* (TWD), launched in 2004, which has been translated into 17 languages and has sold over 1 million copies in Australia.

Manny is a former executive member of the Federal Government Food and Health Dialogue, which influences nutrition reformulation targets for manufactured foods in order to improve the nutritional quality of the Australian food supply. She is also a member of the Heart Foundation Food and Nutrition Advisory Committee, and the Woolworths Healthier Australia Taskforce, among other industry bodies.

Manny is the recipient of three CSIRO Medals, is a Distinguished Alumni of Flinders University, holds a research excellence award from the University of Adelaide and is a recipient of the Zonta Club Woman of International Achievement award.

Megan Rebuli Megan is a research dietitian at CSIRO Health and Biosecurity and an accredited practising dietitian with the Dietitians Association of Australia. She has a background in public health nutrition and epidemiology, as well as experience in dietary assessment and analysis in practice. Megan has worked on clinical trials delivering diet interventions targeting health outcomes including weight loss, cardiovascular disease, and diabetes, as well as enhancing overall health.

Dr Gilly Hendrie Gilly is a research scientist at CSIRO Health and Biosecurity. She has a PhD and expertise in diet, nutrition and obesity prevention. She has worked extensively on the development of new tools to measure dietary intake, and methods to quantify dietary patterns, including the development of indexes to assess diet quality. Gilly has a deep understanding of dietary patterns and how these impact on global concerns such as obesity, food security and climate change. She has published more than 50 peer-reviewed research papers in the areas of nutrition, dietary patterns and lifestyle programs.

Danielle Baird Danielle is a research dietitian at CSIRO Health and Biosecurity. Her expertise lies in analysing dietary data across a number of diverse and complex research areas. Danielle has analysed dietary data from National Nutrition Surveys collected over the past 30 years to gain a comprehensive understanding of Australia's food choices and dietary behaviour, and how these impact on important issues such as obesity, food security, climate change and the need for policy reform.

INTRODUCTION

In 2017, the CSIRO launched *The CSIRO Low-carb Diet*, and the book became a number-one bestseller across Australia. This popularity reflects the enormous shift in focus towards better health within the community.

Some of us are simply looking to lose a few kilos and increase our energy and fitness levels. Others, though, are attempting to manage chronic conditions — including obesity and related metabolic disease such as type 2 diabetes — that interfere dramatically with our quality and enjoyment of life.

What Australians are starting to understand is the extent to which these conditions are caused by the consumption of what may now be regarded as a typical Western diet. This diet is based on the kinds of convenience foods that have been sold to the community as fast and cheap solutions to traditional cooking. Typically, these foods are energy-dense and low in nutrients. It is now well-recognised that the combination of this kind of diet with low levels of exercise and increased time spent in sedentary pursuits (office work, increased screen time, etc) can lead to the development of serious lifestyle diseases.

What sets this low-carb diet apart?

There are many different diets available. If you are reading this book, you have most likely tried a few. Any diet that gets you to eat less will help you lose weight — but not all diets are equal. What is different about the CSIRO Low-carb Diet is that it is not just about short-term weight loss — it's about long-term improvements in our overall health. This is a claim backed by solid scientific evidence from studies conducted by the CSIRO and numerous other top-tier scientific institutions around the world.

For many years, health authorities have told us that fat is bad for us and promoted a diet high in unrefined carbohydrates and low in fat. This has led to the increased consumption of carbohydrate-rich foods such as breads, cereals, rice, pasta, pastries and biscuits, many of which also contain large amounts of sugar. However, nutritional science is constantly evolving. It is now known that high-carbohydrate foods cause rapid elevation of blood-sugar levels which can ultimately lead to type 2 diabetes, heart disease and associated health consequences. It has also become clear that not all fats are equal, and that unsaturated fats — monounsaturated and polyunsaturated fats such as those found in nuts, seeds, oils, avocado and fish — actually improve heart health. Higher intakes of protein also helps people feel full and satisfied after eating.

The CSIRO Low-carb Diet is an energy-controlled diet that significantly reduces carbohydrates while raising the levels of healthy fats and protein through the consumption of nutrient-dense whole foods. This is what differentiates this diet from others — it provides the right balance of carbs, protein and fats; keeps the level of saturated fat low to boost the health-promoting effects; and includes foods from all the major food groups, ensuring the diet is nutritionally complete.

Rigorous scientific evidence shows this diet is not only very effective in promoting substantial weight loss but, compared to a traditional high-carbohydrate, low-fat diet, it improves blood glucose control and normalises blood cholesterol levels, which is particularly beneficial for the treatment of insulin resistance, metabolic syndrome and type 2 diabetes. This research has also shown that, with self-monitoring, this plan and its related health improvements are sustainable over the long term and not a short-lived fad.

Our response to your feedback

Following the publication of *The CSIRO Low-carb Diet*, countless Australians have fallen in love with and adopted this plan to lose weight and improve their health. Doctors and other health practitioners are using this plan in the treatment and management of their patients with great success, as it improves several of the key health targets they measure and are trying to improve. In fact, some people who take medication for high blood pressure, high cholesterol and diabetes may find their need for it reduces significantly as a result of this plan. And because this plan is so effective, readers are encouraged to seek medical advice and undertake the program in close consultation with their healthcare team to maximise the benefits that can be achieved.

This second book has been published in response to the strong demand for this dietary approach and the enormous amount of feedback received from readers, and will be an invaluable companion to the first book. Following the same evidence-based principles and daily food allowances, *CSIRO Low-carb Every Day* provides a wealth of new ideas and greater flexibility to enable you to be more creative in making smart food choices, day in, day out. It includes:

- an update on the latest science
- answers to the most frequently asked questions about low-carb diets
- 80 new delicious recipes with all the daily allowances calculated and explained, and a focus on quick and easy dishes
- meal builders that will help you create your own tasty low-carb recipes using chef-ready food combinations to provide greater flexibility and personalisation while still remaining within the daily food allowances
- a range of new exercises to provide greater variety and interest, including advanced options to ensure you continue to get fitter and stronger.

So many people have tried this plan and had great success. We at the CSIRO hope that you can use this guide to adopt this eating philosophy and lifestyle over the long term, and achieve the significant health benefits and improved quality of life that it can deliver.

WHAT'S DIFFERENT IN THIS BOOK?

The bestselling *CSIRO Low-carb Diet* book introduced many people to this way of eating for the first time. In this book, we're giving you more recipes and exercises, plus lots of flexible food options to help you incorporate the diet into your everyday life.

Quick and easy recipes

In response to feedback from our readers, this book focuses on meals that are simple and quick to prepare, and use fewer ingredients. We understand that many people don't have the time to cook complicated meals, and we wanted to make it as easy as possible to get a nutritious dinner on the table fast. We also wanted to give you options for meals that are easy to transport: food that can be prepped and packed in advance so all you have to do is grab and go.

Eating plans

The first *CSIRO Low-carb Diet* book included 12 weeks' of comprehensive meal plans and exercises to support the diet. In this book, we have provided broader guidelines for you to follow, which give you the tools you need to construct healthy and delicious low-carb meals in any situation.

See pages 28–29 for step-by-step guidelines on how to plan your meals across a day.

- We've created five **day plans** (pages 30–39) that group meals based on a theme and provide the correct units and amount of carbs for a standard 6000 kJ per day. For example, for portable meals to make ahead to take to work, you could turn to page 36 for a 'meals on-the-go' day. Or you could turn to page 38 for a 'vegetarian' day, if you are choosing to go meat-free every now and then.
- Next are the **meal builders** (pages 40–51) which offer ideas on how to construct a meal using the basic food groups. These quick-reference guides show you at a glance which flavours, textures and ingredients go well together, and will help you build your repertoire of go-to dishes. Just choose a meal builder, then use the daily food guide on pages 25–27 to work out the portions required for each food type, taking into account the unit value of your other food choices for that day to ensure you achieve the correct energy requirements for your needs.
- Lastly, our **flavour boosters** (pages 52–57) can help add interest and variety to your cooking. Some of these are grouped into themes based on popular cuisines. These ideas will provide inspiration and give you plenty of options to spice up those everyday foods that form the foundation of this way of eating: low–moderate carb vegetables, lean proteins and healthy fats.

More exercises

On pages 226–239 we have provided new, and in some cases advanced, exercise options that complement those in the first book, to help add variety to your exercise routine, and further improve your fitness, strength and health.

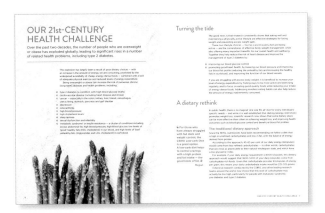

For an overview of the diet and an update on the latest science, turn to pages 6-13.

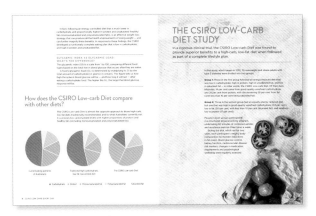

To see how this diet compares to other diets, see page 8.

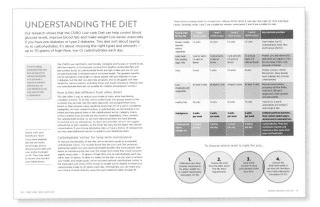

Pages 20-21 are your starting point for working out which level of the diet is best for you.

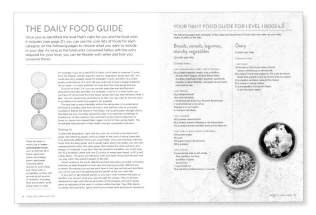

Pages 25-27 list the core foods in each category, to help you choose what you can eat for each meal.

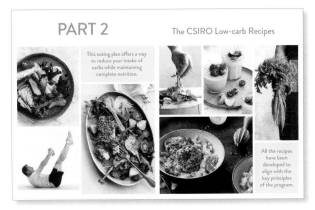

Then turn to page 58 for a collection of delicious, easy-to-make low-carb recipes.

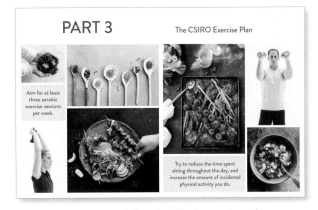

Lastly, see page 226 for detailed exercise plans.

PART 1

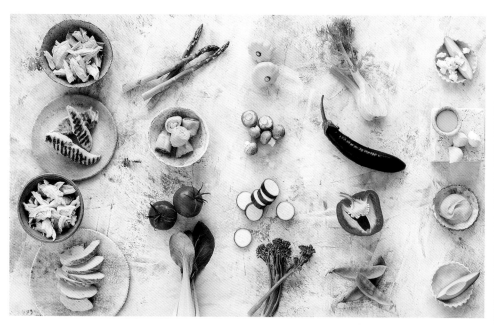

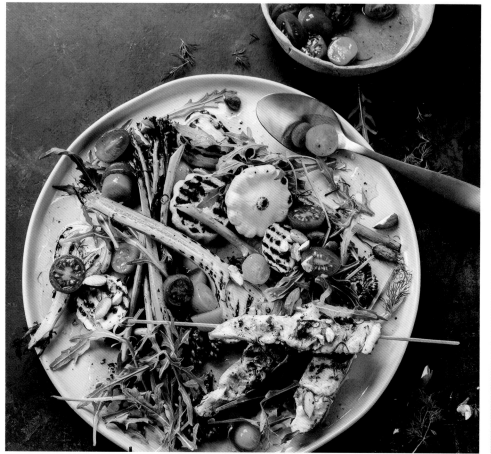

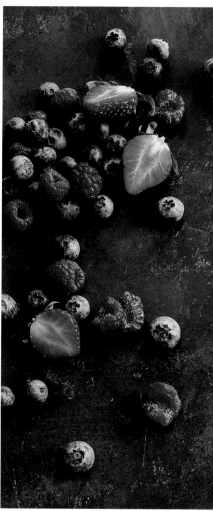

This way
of eating is
nutritionally
complete and
focuses on
whole foods.

Understanding the Low-carb Diet

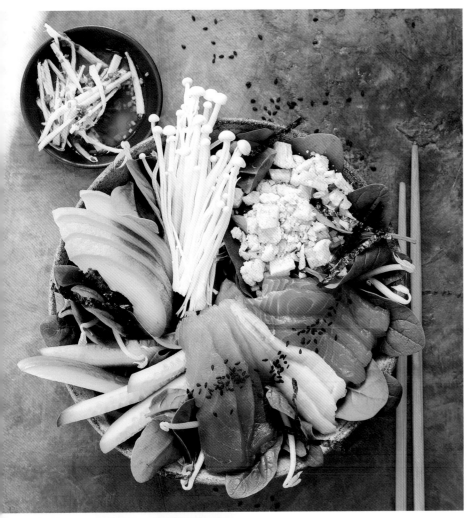

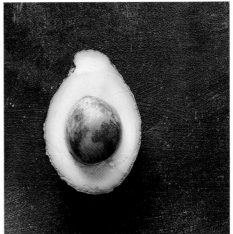

This eating plan is effective for weight loss while also improving your overall health.

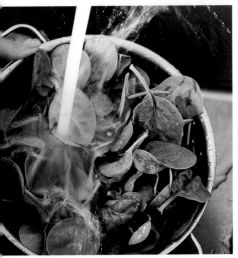

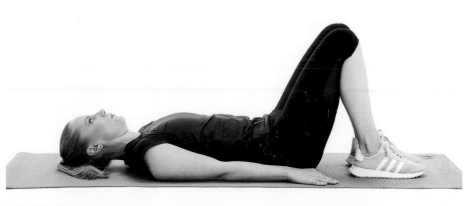

OUR 21st-CENTURY HEALTH CHALLENGE

Over the past two decades, the number of people who are overweight or obese has exploded globally, leading to significant rises in a number of related health problems, including type 2 diabetes.

This explosion has largely been a result of poor dietary choices — with an increase in the amount of energy we are consuming, promoted by the widespread availability of cheap, energy-dense foods — combined with a lack of adequate physical exercise and reduced levels of energy expenditure.

Being overweight or obese can increase the risk of numerous chronic (long-term) diseases and health problems, including:

- type 2 diabetes (a condition with high blood glucose levels)
- cardiovascular disease (including heart disease and stroke)
- cancer — especially in the colon, kidney, liver, breast, oesophagus, uterus lining, stomach, pancreas and gall bladder
- depression
- osteoarthritis
- high blood pressure
- high cholesterol levels
- sleep apnoea
- sexual dysfunction and infertility
- 'metabolic syndrome' or insulin resistance — a cluster of conditions including excess abdominal fat, high blood pressure, high blood glucose, low levels of 'good' healthy fats (HDL cholesterol) in our blood, and high levels of 'bad' unhealthy fats (triglycerides and LDL cholesterol) in our blood.

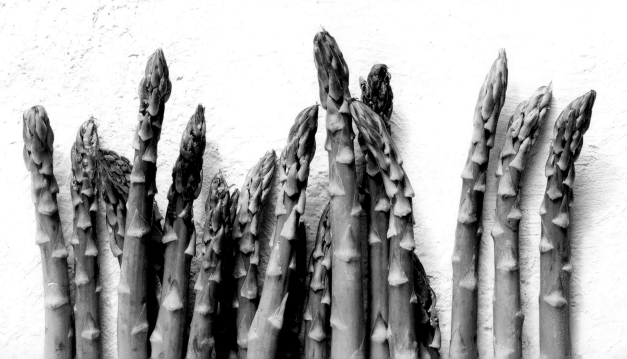

Turning the tide

The good news is that research consistently shows that eating well and maintaining a physically active lifestyle are effective strategies for losing weight and preventing excess weight gain.

These two lifestyle choices — having a good-quality diet and being active — are the cornerstones of effective body-weight management, while also offering many important benefits for our overall health and wellbeing. Together they help reduce the risk of heart disease and improve the management of type 2 diabetes by:

- improving our blood glucose control
- promoting good heart health, by lowering our blood pressure and improving our blood fat profile (reducing the unhealthy fats and increasing the healthy fats in our blood), and improving the function of our blood vessels.

If you are struggling with excess body weight, it is beneficial to increase your level of energy expenditure by finding ways to be more active and exercising regularly, and to focus on eating good-quality foods while reducing your intake of energy-dense foods. Addressing mindless eating habits can also help reduce the amount of energy inadvertently consumed.

A dietary rethink

In public health, there is no magical 'one size fits all' diet for every individual's specific needs — and while it is well established that dieting (energy restriction) promotes weight loss, scientific research now shows that some dietary plans can be more effective than others in achieving weight loss, and improving health outcomes such as blood glucose control and beneficial blood fat profiles.

For those who have always struggled with fad diets and weight control, the CSIRO Low-carb Diet is a great option. A low-carb diet helps to control cravings with a high protein and fat intake — the good kinds of fat.

Megan

The traditional dietary approach

Since the 1970s, nutritionists have been recommending we follow a diet that is high in unrefined carbohydrates and low in fat, with the balance of energy derived from protein.

According to this approach, 45–65 per cent of our daily energy (kilojoules) would come from less-refined carbohydrates — in other words, carbohydrates that are close as practicable to their natural wholegrain state, and which have a low glycaemic index.

For example, if your daily energy requirement is 8000 kilojoules, this dietary approach would suggest that 3600–5200 of your daily kilojoules come from carbohydrate-rich foods. Given that carbohydrate provides 16 kilojoules of energy per gram, this means your daily carbohydrate intake would be 225–325 grams.

Extensive research conducted by the CSIRO, and other leading research teams around the world, now shows that this level of carbohydrate may actually be too high, particularly for people with metabolic syndrome, pre-diabetes and type 2 diabetes.

In fact, following an energy-controlled diet that is much lower in carbohydrate, and proportionally higher in protein and unsaturated 'healthy' fats (monounsaturated and polyunsaturated fats), is an effective weight-loss strategy that can produce all the health improvements of losing weight — *and* can further magnify these benefits. In response to these findings, the CSIRO developed a nutritionally complete eating plan that is low in carbohydrate, and high in protein and unsaturated fat.

GLYCAEMIC INDEX VS GLYCAEMIC LOAD: WHAT'S THE DIFFERENCE?

The glycaemic index (GI) is a scale from 1 to 100, comparing different food types based on the total rise in blood glucose that occurs after they are eaten.

A food's glycaemic load (GL) is determined by multiplying its GI by the total amount of carbohydrate (in grams) it contains. This figure tells us how high the spike in blood glucose will be — and how long it will last — after eating a carbohydrate food. The higher the GL, the larger the blood glucose response will be.

How does the CSIRO Low-carb Diet compare with other diets?

The CSIRO Low-carb Diet is almost the opposite approach to those high-carb, low-fat diets traditionally recommended, and to what Australians currently eat. It combines low carbohydrate levels with higher proportions of protein and healthy fats (including monounsaturated and polyunsaturated fat).

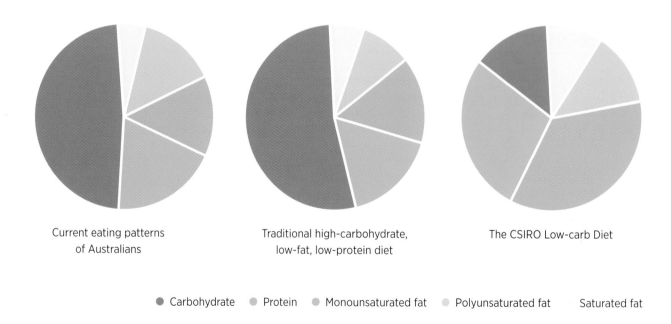

Current eating patterns of Australians

Traditional high-carbohydrate, low-fat, low-protein diet

The CSIRO Low-carb Diet

● Carbohydrate   ● Protein   ● Monounsaturated fat   ● Polyunsaturated fat   ● Saturated fat

THE CSIRO LOW-CARB DIET STUDY

In a rigorous clinical trial, the CSIRO Low-carb Diet was found to provide superior benefits to a high-carb, low-fat diet when followed as part of a complete lifestyle plan.

In this study, which began in 2012, 115 overweight and obese adults with type 2 diabetes were divided into two groups.

Group 1: Those in the first group followed an energy-reduced diet that was low in carbohydrate, high in protein, high in unsaturated fat, and low in saturated fat — in other words, the CSIRO Low-carb Diet. Of their daily kilojoules, 14 per cent came from good-quality unrefined carbohydrate, and 28 per cent from protein, with the remaining 58 per cent from fat (with less than 10 per cent being saturated fat).

Group 2: Those in the second group had an equally energy-reduced diet, but one that was high in good-quality unrefined carbohydrate (53 per cent), low in fat (30 per cent, with less than 10 per cent saturated fat), and relatively low in protein (17 per cent).

People in both groups participated in a structured physical activity program, undertaking 60 minutes of combined aerobic and resistance exercise three times a week.

During the trial, which ran for two years, each participant's weight, body composition (to monitor reductions in fat mass), blood glucose control, kidney function, cardiovascular disease risk markers, changes in medication requirements and psychological wellbeing were regularly assessed.

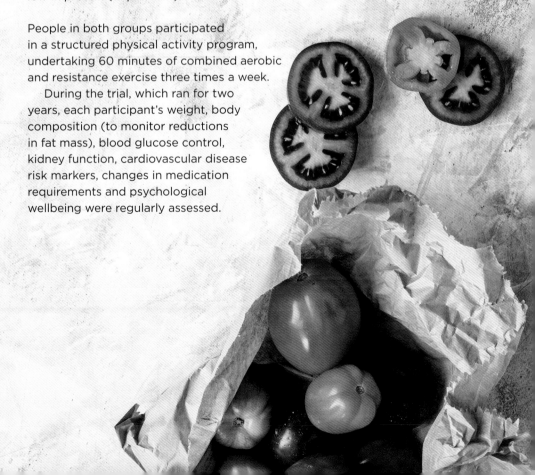

One-year results

After 12 months, the number of people who remained in the study was similar between the groups: 41 people (71 per cent) from the low-carb group and 37 people (65 per cent) from the high-carb group.

While both groups enjoyed substantial reductions in body weight, fat mass and blood pressure, as well as improved mood and quality of life, there were striking differences between the two diet groups in terms of several important health outcomes — as the table below shows.

The low-carb group experienced much greater reductions in their need for diabetes medication — a reduction that was **twice as large** as in the high-carb group. Also, in the low-carb group, the improvement in daily glycaemic stability (blood sugar control) was **three times** that in the high-carb group. Better blood sugar control means a lower risk of hypoglycaemia, reduced medication costs, and fewer medication side effects.

Blood triglycerides ('bad' unhealthy fats) also decreased more on the low-carb diet, with a higher increase in HDL ('good' healthy) cholesterol — which equated to a 24 per cent decrease in their cardiovascular disease risk.

Benefits enjoyed by both diet groups

Health measure	Average change in the low-carb diet group	Average change in the high-carb group
Body weight	–9.1% (10 kg)	–9.1% (10 kg)
Fat mass	–8.3 kg	–8.3 kg
Systolic/diastolic blood pressure	–6/6 mmHg	–6/6 mmHg
HbA1c	–1% (-12.6 mmol/mol)	–1% (-12.6 mmol/mol)
Fasting glucose	–1.4 mmol/L	–1.4 mmol/L
LDL cholesterol	–0.1 mmol/L	–0.2 mmol/L
Mood and quality of life	about 30% improvement	about 30% improvement

Both groups enjoyed substantial reductions in body weight, fat mass, blood pressure, HbA1c and fasting glucose, as well as improved mood and quality of life.

Significant extra benefits of the low-carb diet group

Health measure	Average change in the low-carb diet group	Average change in the high-carb group
Medication requirements*	–40%	–20%
Glycaemic variability	–30%	–10%
Blood triglycerides	–0.4 mmol/L	–0.01 mmol/L
HDL cholesterol	+0.1 mmol/L	+0.06 mmol/L

*Medications for controlling blood glucose levels

Two years on...

Since the release of *The CSIRO Low-carb Diet*, research into the diet has been continuing.

After completing the first 52 weeks of the two-year CSIRO clinical trial, study participants continued for a further 12 months, with follow-up assessments performed again after two years. These results have now been analysed and published.

After two years, the number of people who completed the trial remained similar between both groups: 33 people (57%) from the low-carb group, compared with 28 people (49%) from the high-carb group. Importantly, the benefits and differences in the health outcomes between the groups were maintained after two years.

These findings show that both dietary patterns studied in the trial are equally sustainable and can be followed over the long term to achieve significant health benefits, and that the superior health advantages of the low-carb diet can be maintained. However, and importantly, this study also indicates that the low-carb approach can offer **significant extra long-term benefits** for people with metabolic syndrome, pre-diabetes and type 2 diabetes.

Other emerging published research further supports our findings and the benefit of carbohydrate-restricted diets in people with type 2 diabetes. A recent meta-analysis — a combined analytical summary of multiple good-quality clinical trials that have been conducted by distinguished research groups around the world — showed that compared to a high-carb, low-fat diet, consuming a diet with a low to moderate amount of carbohydrate had greater effects on improving blood glucose control in people with type 2 diabetes. Indeed, this meta-analysis further showed that the greater the level of carbohydrate restriction, the greater the improvement in blood glucose control.

This recent meta-analysis further supports our clinical findings that the CSIRO Low-carb Diet is effective for weight loss, while also improving your health.

Why the CSIRO Low-carb Diet works

There are several reasons why the CSIRO Low-carb Diet approach is so effective in helping you lose excess weight, while also making you feel better and significantly improving your metabolic and cardiovascular health.

It reduces your glycaemic load

While selecting foods with a low glycaemic index reduces the glycaemic load of your meals, having a **lower total amount of carbohydrate** is what actually has the greatest effect on reducing the overall glycaemic load of your diet.

A lower glycaemic load reduces your blood glucose response after a meal or snack, making it easier to achieve more stable blood glucose levels throughout the day.

The **higher proportion of protein and healthy fats** in the CSIRO Low-carb Diet helps to further blunt rises in blood glucose levels after carbohydrate is consumed. Again, this helps reduce blood glucose spikes and fluctuations, and improves blood glucose control through the day.

GL

↓

GI/100

×

Total amount of
carbohydrate
eaten (grams)

You don't feel as hungry

The **higher protein intake** also helps you feel fuller for longer, suppressing
your appetite. This reduces the desire to snack throughout the day, giving
you better control of your energy intake, making it easier for you to maintain
a lower body weight.

You burn more energy

Digesting and absorbing food accounts for about 10 per cent of our daily
energy expenditure. It takes more energy to digest protein, compared to
carbohydrate or fat — so having a **higher proportion of protein** in the diet
actually helps you expend more energy throughout the day.

Also, on the CSIRO Low-carb Diet, the higher amounts of protein can
increase the proportion of weight loss from fat reserves, allowing you to
retain more fat-free mass and muscle. Even when we're at rest, our muscles
require fuel to keep working, which is what largely drives our individual
resting metabolic rate — so by maintaining a higher muscle and fat-free
mass on our higher-protein weight-loss diet, our bodies are expending more
energy throughout the day and when we are sleeping. Having a higher resting
metabolic rate can help us maintain a lower body weight over the long term.

This effect can be further magnified by combining a higher-protein diet
with **increased physical exercise**, particularly resistance or strength-training
exercise, which is part of the exercise plan in this book (see pages 226–239).
An appropriate level of physical activity is an important factor in weight loss
and weight maintenance, as well as improved overall health.

More muscle mass also means better glucose control

Muscle is one of the body's major storage sites for glucose, so maintaining
a **larger muscle mass** makes it easier for your body to transport and store
glucose from the blood. This is helpful for fighting 'insulin resistance', and
achieving good blood glucose control — which is particularly important for
people with metabolic syndrome, pre-diabetes or type 2 diabetes.

It's high in good fats to keep you healthy

The CSIRO diet has a higher proportion of unsaturated 'healthy' fats, including
monounsaturated and polyunsaturated fats.

Unsaturated fats can reduce your risk of type 2 diabetes by improving
insulin sensitivity, producing a lower blood glucose response after meals.

Unsaturated fats also reduce your risk of cardiovascular disease by:

- increasing the 'good' HDL (high-density lipoprotein) cholesterol in your blood,
which picks up excess cholesterol in your blood and takes it back to your liver,
where it is broken down and removed from your body
- reducing levels of 'bad' LDL (low-density lipoprotein) cholesterol, as well
as total cholesterol and triglycerides — the blood fats that can lead to
atherosclerosis (hardening and narrowing of the arteries)
- improving the functioning of the blood vessels in the heart.

Rich sources of **monounsaturated fats** include avocados, nuts and seeds,
olive oil and canola oil, lean fish and chicken, and olives.

Good sources of **polyunsaturated fats** include fish (particularly salmon
and sardines), nuts and seeds, sunflower oil and sesame oil, and soy beans.

It has plenty of fibre

Unlike some low-carb, high-protein diets, the CSIRO eating plan delivers the **recommended daily fibre intake** of 25–30 grams — mainly from generous quantities of low-carb vegetables, but also a small amount of high-fibre grains and legumes.

An adequate daily fibre intake is important not only for gut and bowel health, but also helps us feel more satisfied and replete after meals so we are less likely to overeat.

It is nutritionally balanced and sustainable

Unlike some diets, which can leave you feeling washed out, tired and depleted, the CSIRO Low-carb Diet provides adequate intakes of all the essential vitamins, minerals and trace elements needed for good health.

In fact, after two years we assessed people's blood status levels of **key vitamins and minerals** including vitamin B12, folate, beta-carotene, vitamin D, vitamin E, copper, zinc, selenium, calcium, magnesium, sodium, potassium and iron. The results showed that the average levels of these nutrients were within the normal (laboratory-specific) reference ranges for both groups following either the CSIRO Low-carb Diet and the traditional high-carb, low-fat diet.

As well as significantly improving people's physical health, our clinical trial found that following the CSIRO Low-carb Diet and exercise plan markedly improved people's **psychological mood** and perceived quality of life, meaning they were more likely to stick with the program.

Offering a sustainable approach to weight management, the CSIRO Low-carb Diet and exercise plan can be maintained over the long term, as part of a healthy lifestyle.

If you're vegetarian, or have specific food preferences or a history of nutritional deficiencies, a dietitian can help tailor the diet to ensure you are getting all the nutrients you need.

> ❝ The recipes in this book have been invaluable to me. They are delicious and, most importantly, very satisfying, which has helped with reducing my cravings for carbs and has led to steady weight loss. ❞
>
> *Danielle*

Before you begin...

Because the CSIRO Low-carb Diet plan can be so effective in improving a range of health measures, we recommend you see your GP before starting this diet, and that they regularly check your blood pressure, blood glucose and blood cholesterol levels once you begin the diet.

This is a good opportunity to have your GP update your medical, family and lifestyle history — particularly if you have not had a review within the previous two years — and to build a relationship with your doctor, so they can help support your journey on the plan.

This is particularly important if you are taking medications to control your blood pressure, blood glucose and/or blood cholesterol levels, because chances are that your level of medications may need to be reduced as a result of following this plan.

We also urge you to familiarise your healthcare team with the principles of the CSIRO Low-carb Diet plan — including your dietitian, exercise physiologist, and psychologist, if required — so they can also assist you in improving your overall health.

CSIRO LOW-CARB DIET: FREQUENTLY ASKED QUESTIONS

In addition to the high level of positive feedback we have received in response to our previous book, *The CSIRO Low-carb Diet,* we have also received letters and emails from readers asking about certain aspects of the diet. The most common ones are answered below.

❶ Why is the diet low in saturated fat?

Some low-carbohydrate diets, as well as increasing the overall proportion of dietary fat consumed, also promote a high intake of saturated fat.

In comparison, while the CSIRO Low-carb Diet also increases the intake of dietary fat, it does so by increasing the amount of **unsaturated ('healthy') fats**, while limiting saturated fat to no more than 10 per cent of total daily energy intake. This amount of saturated fat is consistent with national dietary recommendations.

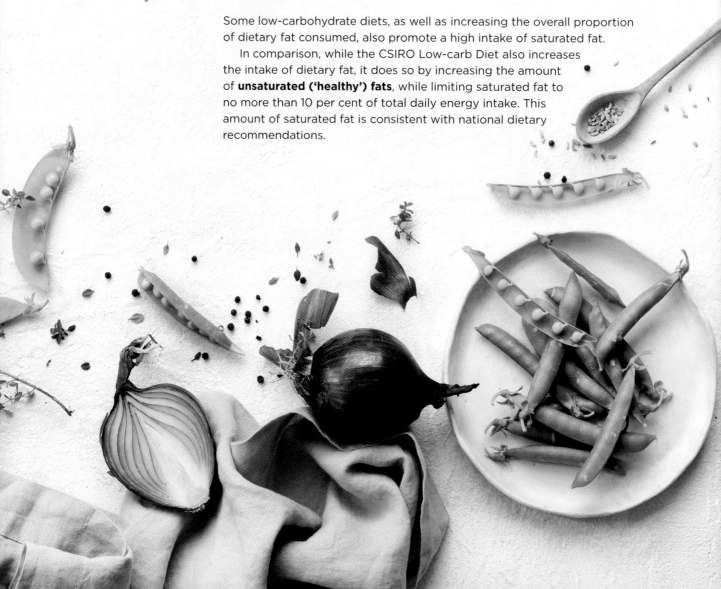

It is true that scientific evidence continues to evolve, and there is growing debate about whether saturated fat is bad for us — and whether it's as closely linked to increasing the risk of heart disease and type 2 diabetes as previously thought.

Nevertheless, a large body of scientific research shows that a high intake of saturated fat can increase a number of risk factors for heart disease and type 2 diabetes, including:

- promoting insulin resistance
- elevating LDL ('bad') cholesterol levels, which leads to atherosclerosis
- impairing blood vessel function, particularly in the heart, which can increase the risk of heart disease.

In fact, our clinical research has shown that a low-carb diet that was high in saturated fat actually increased LDL cholesterol levels, and also impaired blood vessel function, compared to a traditional low-fat diet that was high in unrefined carbohydrates.

In contrast, when we compared a CSIRO Low-carb-style Diet — a **low-carb** diet **high in unsaturated 'healthy' fat** and **low in saturated fat** — with a low-fat diet high in unrefined carbs, both diets had similar responses in LDL cholesterol levels and blood vessel function, with little difference between them.

This evidence suggests it is still a good idea to replace foods high in saturated fat with small amounts of foods containing unsaturated fat. In fact, a published systematic review that summarises the results of over 100 well-controlled dietary intervention studies conducted in humans has shown that increasing the intake of healthy fats (monounsaturated fat and polyunsaturated fat) in place of carbohydrate and saturated fat can improve blood glucose control and reduce insulin resistance.

This is why the CSIRO Low-carb Diet limits the saturated fat content to no more than 10 per cent of total daily energy intake — to capitalise on these health advantages.

❷ Why does the diet recommend low-fat dairy options?

While debate continues on the effects of high saturated fat intake on increasing the risk of heart disease and type 2 diabetes (see above), research indicates that the saturated fat contained in most dairy foods does not appear to increase heart disease risk. Nevertheless, the CSIRO Low-carb Diet has been comprehensively designed to consider the overall nutrient balance, as well as the total calorie count. Using **low-fat dairy options** ensures the dietary plan promotes effective weight loss and achieves health improvements while remaining nutritionally complete, delivering all the essential vitamins and minerals, in particular dietary calcium.

If you prefer the taste of regular-fat dairy, you can still enjoy it on this eating plan — just keep in mind that this may increase your total energy intake. See page 25 for guidelines on portion sizes allowed.

❸ Do active individuals need extra carbs?

To meet our energy needs between meals — whether we're at rest or undertaking physical activity — the body is able to draw upon stored fat, as well as the limited amount of glucose that is stored in our liver and muscles in the form of glycogen.

During rest (e.g. sitting or lying down) and low-intensity physical activity (such as slow walking), our bodies use mostly stored fat for energy.

As our exercise intensity increases, a greater proportion of our energy needs are drawn from glycogen, which can be broken down more quickly to produce energy, compared to fat.

Our bodies typically store enough glycogen (around 8000 kilojoules) to fuel about 60–120 minutes of vigorous exercise (such as jogging, running and lap swimming), and much longer sessions of moderate-intensity exercise (such as brisk walking and doubles tennis).

If our glycogen becomes depleted, this can cause sudden fatigue, or what athletes refer to as 'hitting the wall'. When carbohydrate is consumed, it is converted to glucose, which is used as an immediate fuel source for exercise, and also to replenish glycogen stores. Once glycogen stores have been fully replenished, surplus glucose is converted into fat.

For most of us it is not necessary

Some people believe that a high-carbohydrate diet is necessary to maintain sufficient muscle glycogen to sustain a **healthy, active lifestyle**, and to participate in regular physical activity and vigorous exercise. However, for most of us this is not the case, as we are unlikely to exercise for a sufficient duration, intensity and frequency to deplete our glycogen stores — even when we consume a reduced amount of carbohydrate during the day.

Furthermore, when consuming a low-carbohydrate diet, within days our bodies begin to adapt, to increase the proportion of fat used for fuel during both rest and exercise. In fact, some evidence suggests this improved fat-burning capacity may even help to better preserve muscle glycogen, and enable us to perform endurance activity for longer.

This means that most people do not require carbohydrate during exercise, and most people on a low-carb diet do not experience any sustained negative effects on their physical performance, or on their ability to participate in regular moderate-intensity exercise.

Indeed, when we assessed adult men and women from the general population, our research showed there were **no differences** in their maximal aerobic fitness, muscle strength, ability to perform or perception of fatigue, while they were undertaking a regular moderate-intensity exercise program — regardless of whether they were on a high-carb diet or a low-carb diet.

Very elite endurance athletes may need a little extra

Of course, there may be some exceptions for special populations such as elite endurance athletes, whose exercise levels and performance targets are significantly higher than those of the general population. Athletes who undertake high volumes of exercise training, or perform exercise at very high intensities, and/or for extended periods — such as those who compete in marathons, or have frequent back-to-back intensive training sessions throughout the day — are at greater risk of depleting the body's muscle glycogen stores, and may therefore need to consume some additional carbohydrate before, during and/or after exercise to avoid 'hitting the wall'.

There is also limited evidence that the increased utilisation of fuel from fat that occurs when following a low-carb diet may negatively affect the race-day performance of an elite endurance athlete.

However, these issues will not be relevant for most of the population. If you are an elite endurance athlete, an accredited sports dietitian will be able to tailor your individual carbohydrate requirements for your exercise needs.

④ What if I'm on medication or have medical issues?

As we have seen, there are many benefits that can be gained from following the CSIRO Low-carb Diet and lifestyle plan.

However, before embarking on any new lifestyle plan that will alter your diet or change your exercise routine, it is important to **talk with your GP** and healthcare team — particularly if you have a current medical condition, are taking medications, are unsure if a low-carb diet is right for you, or have undergone a surgical procedure that may impact on your food choices or tolerance to certain foods.

Your healthcare team will be able to tailor the plan to suit your personal needs, and also monitor your health as you make changes to your lifestyle, to help you get the most out of the CSIRO Low-carb Diet plan.

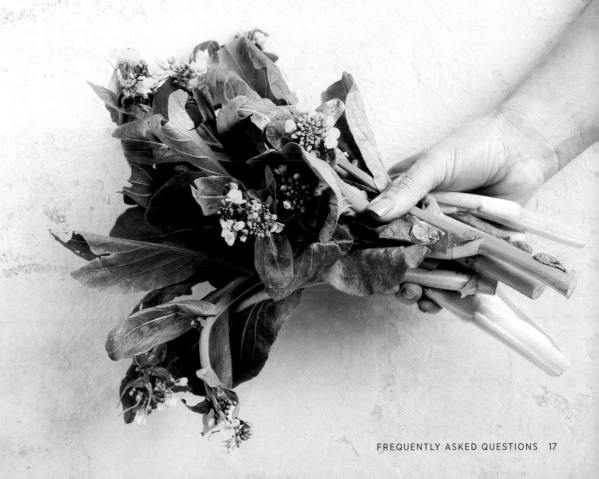

⑤ Is fruit still allowed?

While you can eat as many non-starchy, low-carbohydrate vegetables as you like on this plan, fruit intake has been restricted. This is because of its high sugar content in the form of fructose, which is broken down to glucose and released into the bloodstream, causing blood glucose to rise sharply.

Fruit is still allowed but restricted. Many of the nutrients fruits provide are also found in vegetables, so this isn't a problem. However, you can enjoy fruit in exchange for another carbohydrate-based food, to help balance your total carbohydrate intake for the day.

If you are at the maintenance stage of the diet, namely from week 7 onwards, here's a guide to the serving quantity of different fruits you can enjoy to obtain your extra carb portion.

CARBOHYDRATE EXTRAS	1 serving = 1 carb extra (10 g carb or less)
FRESH FRUIT — choose most	
Apples	50 g
Apricots	2 medium
Bananas	40 g
Blueberries, frozen or fresh	60 g
Cherries	60 g
Feijoa	3
Figs	2
Kiwifruit	2 small
Lemon or lime juice, freshly squeezed	300 ml (can add to sparkling water)
Nectarine	1 small
Oranges	100 g
Passionfruit	7 (100 g)
Passionfruit pulp (no syrup)	50 g
Peach	1 small
Pears	50 g
Persimmon	1 small
Raspberries, frozen or fresh	100 g
Rhubarb (stewed, no added sugar)	400 g
Strawberries	200 g
DRIED FRUIT — choose least	
Apricots	20 g
Dates	2
Figs	1 (20 g)
Mixed dried fruit	10 g
Sultanas	10 g

⑥ What drinks are allowed on the Low-carb Diet?

When following the CSIRO Low-carb Diet, you will need to minimise your consumption of fruit drinks and sugar-sweetened beverages such as soft drinks, sports drinks and sweetened milks — or better still, avoid them altogether.

Many of these drinks are **high in carbohydrate** and often contain added refined sugar, which can make blood glucose rise sharply, and also contribute extra kilojoules to your daily intake for minimal nutritional value.

However, you can enjoy a range of suitable alternatives, including:

- naturally flavoured mineral water
- mineral or soda water flavoured with a slice of lemon or lime, or strawberries or mint leaves
- diet soft drinks, diet cordial or diet soda stream
- tea, including herbal teas — no added sugar, and with any milk used being part of the daily dairy allocation (50 ml = ¼ unit)
- coffee — no added sugar, and with any milk used being part of the daily dairy allocation (50 ml = ¼ unit).

See pages 224–225 for suggestions of suitable drinks allowed on the diet.

Alcoholic drinks are part of the optional indulgence allowance, comprising two serves a week. A single indulgence would be 100 ml wine or 30 ml spirits.

⑦ How do I maintain the diet in the long term?

Maintaining motivation — especially in the early stages of a new eating and exercise plan — is one of the areas in which some people may need a bit of extra support. That is why we've designed this book so that it can also be used in conjunction with a variety of care providers who can offer you the individual support you may need. Take this book with you to your healthcare provider. They will be able to help personalise strategies for **longer-term maintenance**.

- An accredited practising dietitian can help you find ways to implement this diet pattern. For more information, see **daa.asn.au/what-dietitans-do**.
- A psychologist can help you with any emotional issues that may be contributing to food cravings or unhealthy eating patterns. To find one near you, visit **psychology.org.au/findapsychologist**.
- An accredited exercise physiologist can help you start and stay motivated on an exercise program, and tailor the program to your specific needs. You'll find more information at **essa.org.au/find-aep**.

UNDERSTANDING THE DIET

Our research shows that the CSIRO Low-carb Diet can help control blood glucose levels, improve blood fats and make weight loss easier, especially if you have pre-diabetes or type 2 diabetes. This diet isn't about saying *no* to carbohydrates, it's about choosing the right types and amounts — up to 70 grams of high-fibre, low-GI carbohydrates each day.

> If you're taking medication that may have an impact on nutrient absorption or if you have a history of nutrient deficiencies, see your dietitian as you may need to take a supplement.

Check with your healthcare team

If you have diabetes and are on insulin, we strongly advise discussing the diet with your endocrinologist or GP. They may need to review and monitor your medications.

The CSIRO Low-carb Diet is nutritionally complete and focuses on whole foods, with the majority of its kilojoules coming from healthy unsaturated fats and lean protein foods. Its carbohydrate foods are high in fibre and low-GI, and include foods high in resistant starch for bowel health. The greatest benefits can be enjoyed by overweight or obese people with pre-diabetes or type 2 diabetes, but the diet can also help all adults who've struggled with their weight for various reasons, including those with insulin resistance. (Please note: low-carbohydrate diets are not suitable for children and pregnant women.)

How is this diet different from other diets?

This diet offers a way to reduce your intake of carbs while maintaining complete nutrition. To do this, we've sorted foods into groups based on the nutrients they provide (see the table opposite), and assigned them units based on their kilojoule value (anything lower than 0.5 of a unit is considered negligible). As fruits contain fructose, a carbohydrate, we recommend a low intake and have placed them in the carbohydrate 'extras' category (many of the nutrients fruits provide are also found in vegetables). Dairy contains the carbohydrate lactose, so we have reduced portions but have allowed for almond and soy alternatives. As dairy also provides calcium, we suggest reduced-fat or skim varieties, as the lower the dairy fat the higher the calcium concentration. If you choose alternative dairy or have a history of osteoporosis, you may need additional calcium so speak to your healthcare team.

Carbohydrate 'extras' for long-term maintenance

To improve the flexibility of the diet, we've devised a guide to acceptable carbohydrate 'extras'. Our studies found that the Low-carb Diet produced substantial weight loss and optimised health benefits. But some people were better at maintaining the diet *over the longer term* when they could consume slightly more carbs — 70 grams of high-fibre, low-GI carbohydrates each day, rather than 50 grams. So after six weeks on the diet, or as you start to achieve your health and weight goals, we've included optional carbohydrate 'extras' in the meal plans and some of the recipes to enable you to slightly increase your carbohydrate intake by 20 grams each day. Alternatively, you can make your own choice of extra carbs by using the quick-reference table on page 18.

There are four energy levels to choose from, offering 6000–9000 kJ per day, that cater for most individual needs. Generally, levels 1 and 2 are suitable for women, while levels 3 and 4 are suitable for men.

Food groups for the diet	Level 1 (6000 kJ/day)	Level 2 (7000 kJ/day)	Level 3 (8000 kJ/day)	Level 4 (9000 kJ/day)	Key nutrients provided
Breads, cereals, legumes, starchy vegetables	1.5 units	1.5 units	1.5 units	1.5 units	Slow-release, low-GI, carbohydrates, folate, fibre and B-group vitamins.
Lean meat, fish, poultry, eggs, tofu	1 unit at lunch, 1.5 units at dinner	1 unit at lunch, 2 units at dinner	1 unit at lunch, 2.5 units at dinner	1.5 units at lunch, 2.5 units at dinner	Protein, zinc and vitamin B12. Red meats are highest in iron, fish in omega-3 fatty acids and pork in thiamin.
Dairy	3 units	3 units	3.5 units	4 units	Protein, calcium, vitamin B12 and zinc. Dairy (except most cheeses) also contains carbohydrates.
Low-moderate carb vegetables	At least 5 units	At least 5 units	At least 5 units	At least 5 units	Minimal carbohydrates, and plenty of fibre, folate, vitamins A, B6 and C, magnesium, beta-carotene and antioxidants.
Healthy fats	10 units	11 units	14 units	15 units	Vitamins A, E and K, antioxidants and omega-3 and omega-6 fats.
Indulgences	**2 units per week**	**2 units per week**	**2 units per week**	**2 units per week**	**Limited beneficial nutrients. Most contain added sugars, alcohol and/or saturated fats.**
Carbohydrate extras (Weeks 7+)	**2 extras per day**	**2 extras per day**	**2 extras per day**	**2 extras per day**	**Carbohydrates. They also contribute vitamins and minerals as they come from your core food units.**

To choose which level is right for you...

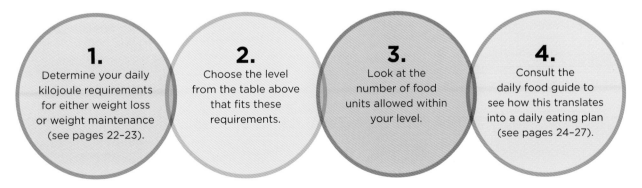

1. Determine your daily kilojoule requirements for either weight loss or weight maintenance (see pages 22–23).

2. Choose the level from the table above that fits these requirements.

3. Look at the number of food units allowed within your level.

4. Consult the daily food guide to see how this translates into a daily eating plan (see pages 24–27).

Determining your daily kilojoule requirements

The following calculation was used in our scientific trial to personalise the diet to each participant's energy needs. It estimates your daily kilojoule requirements to maintain normal body function and keep your weight stable. This is known as your basal metabolic rate (BMR). To determine your BMR, use the appropriate formula from the table below.

Formulas for calculating your basal metabolic rate

Age (years)	BMR equation	
	Women	Men
18–29	(62 x weight in kilograms) + 2036	(63 x weight in kilograms) + 2896
30–59	(34 x weight in kilograms) + 3538	(48 x weight in kilograms) + 3653
60 and over	(38 x weight in kilograms) + 2755	(49 x weight in kilograms) + 2459

Note: There are a few different methods for calculating BMR. We've used the Schofield equation.

Once you've determined your BMR, you need to multiply it by an activity factor from the table below to estimate your total daily kilojoule requirements.

Activity factors for determining your total daily kilojoule requirements

Activity level	Description	Activity factor	
		Women	Men
Sedentary	Very physically inactive (work and leisure)	1.3	1.3
Lightly active	Daily activity of walking or intense exercise once or twice a week and a sedentary job	1.5	1.6
Moderately active	Intense exercise lasting 20–45 minutes at least three times a week or an active job with a lot of daily walking	1.6	1.7
Very active	Intense exercise lasting at least one hour each day or a heavy, physical job	1.9	2.1
Extremely active	Daily intense activity (i.e. nonstop training, e.g. an athlete in training) or a highly demanding physical job (e.g. armed forces)	2.2	2.4

If you're a healthy weight, there's no need to reduce your energy intake, so the number you're left with now is your daily requirement, and you can use this to choose the level from the table on page 21.

If you need to lose weight, calculate your daily kilojoule requirement as follows. To reduce your weight by about 0.5 kilogram each week, you'll need to reduce your energy intake by 2000 kJ per day. Once you've calculated your total daily kilojoule requirements above, subtract 2000 from this number to determine how many kilojoules to eat each day to achieve weight loss, and therefore which of the four levels to choose.

To reduce your weight by about 1 kilogram each week, you'll need to reduce your energy intake by 4000 kJ per day. Calculate your total daily kilojoule needs as above and subtract 4000. This will tell you how many kilojoules to eat each day to achieve this weight loss and therefore which of the four levels to choose.

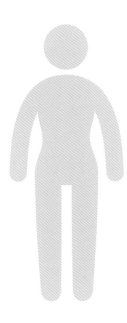

How it works in practice

Sylvia is 58 years old and weighs 87 kilograms. She works part time as an office assistant and looks after her grandchildren two days a week. Sylvia goes for a walk most days. This makes her activity factor 1.5. She chooses the appropriate formula from the table opposite and calculates her BMR like this:

BMR = (34 x weight in kilograms) + 3538
    = (34 x 87) + 3538
    = 6496 kJ per day

To calculate her total daily kilojoule requirements, Sylvia will multiply her BMR by her activity factor:

Total daily energy requirement = 6496 x 1.5
                                    = 9744 kJ per day

This is the amount of energy Sylvia needs to maintain her current weight.

Sylvia is overweight and would like to start by losing about 0.5 kilogram a week. She'll therefore reduce her estimated total daily kilojoule intake by 2000 kJ per day:

Total dieting energy requirement   = 9744 – 2000
                                        = 7744 kJ per day

Sylvia rounds this down to the nearest thousand, 7000 kJ per day, and will therefore start on level 2. If she's feeling too hungry or losing weight too rapidly, Sylvia can move to level 3 (8000 kJ). If she's not losing weight, she can drop down to level 1 (6000 kJ).

Our clinical experience has shown that if your calculated energy requirements are greater than 9000 kJ a day, even by 2000–3000 kJ, following the level 4 diet will still result in significant health benefits.

Maintenance in the longer term

Sylvia reaches her weight-loss goal after six weeks, and her health has improved significantly. She decides she's enjoying the diet but would like to eat some fruit each day. As she's now on maintenance, she can have up to 70 grams carbohydrates each day, instead of the standard 50 grams. To add another carbohydrate serve, she uses the carbohydrate exchange table on page 18 to select a fruit portion.

See how you progress — if your chosen level isn't working, you can move between levels until you start to see the changes you desire. Many people hit a weight-loss plateau after an initial drop in weight. If this happens, you can simply switch to a lower level until you reach your target. Your dietitian and exercise physiologist can also help you overcome a weight plateau.

THE DAILY FOOD GUIDE

Once you've identified the level that's right for you and the food units it includes (see page 21), you can use the core lists of foods for each category on the following pages to choose what you want to include in your day. As long as the total units consumed tallies with the units required for your level, you can be flexible with when and how you consume these.

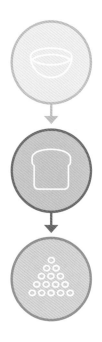

There has been a recent rise in **lower-carbohydrate foods**, such as Herman Brot bread, pasta and cereal, and Helga's lower-carb bread. Choosing these options as your bread and cereal units is acceptable, as they still provide good sources of nutrients, including fibre and protein, while being lower in carbs.

For example, if you're on the 6000 kJ level, you'll need to consume 1.5 units from the 'Breads, cereals, legumes, starchy vegetables' group each day. You could have 30 g suitable cereal for breakfast (1 unit), and then 50 g sweet potato at dinnertime (0.5 unit) OR you could opt to have a bigger breakfast (45 g cereal = 1.5 units) and then no more from this food group that day.

If you're on levels 2–4, you can use this base plan and add the extra allowances your plan provides. For example, if you're on a level 3 plan, you can have 0.5 serve more from the 'Dairy' group each day than the base (level 1) plan. You can choose how you'd like to do this: you may want to have an extra 10 g cheese or an extra 50 g yoghurt, for example.

The best way to enjoy flexibility within the eating plan is to understand the foods it includes; start with the basics and add new ones as you build confidence. Before the research trial began, many participants thought they'd feel deprived, but once they started the diet, most reported no feelings of missing out. On the contrary, they said that having a narrow selection of foods to choose from helped them regain control of their eating habits. The remarkable improvement in their health was also a powerful motivator.

Easing in

To eliminate temptation, start with the core lists of foods in the daily food guide (see following pages) until you adapt to the style of eating, especially if it's drastically different from your usual intake. Once you're familiar with the foods from the daily guide, which usually takes about two weeks, you can start swapping foods within the same group that contain the same nutrients and energy. For example, if you don't feel like cereal for breakfast, you could swap the 30 g breakfast cereal with one 35 g slice of mixed grain bread, or 80 g red kidney beans. This gives you flexibility with your food choices but ensures that you stay within the nutrient targets of the diet.

When looking at the foods selected and the daily plans provided, remember that they've been designed so that each food group provides different key nutrients. By making sure you eat each food in the type and amount specified, you can be sure you'll be gaining the full benefit of the Low-carb Diet.

If you want to get started quickly or you don't wish to follow the plans or builders, you can just work your way through the recipes. They've all been developed to align with the key principles of the program, and each recipe gives an indication of the units it contains within the plan. They offer plenty of variety, and use herbs, spices and nuts to create taste and texture sensations.

YOUR DAILY FOOD GUIDE FOR LEVEL 1 (6000 kJ)

The following pages give examples of the types and quantities of foods that can make up your daily intake of units on the diet.

Breads, cereals, legumes, starchy vegetables

1.5 units per day

Choose from:

1 UNIT HIGH-SOLUBLE-FIBRE, LOW-GI CEREALS

30 g suitable breakfast cereals, such as All-Bran, All-Bran Fibre Toppers, All-Bran Wheat Flakes, Goodness Superfoods Heart, Goodness Superfoods Digestive, Hi-Bran Weet-Bix, untoasted natural muesli, raw (natural) oats

1 UNIT BREADS

35 g multigrain bread

1 thin slice fruit bread

½ wholemeal pita bread (e.g. Mountain Bread wrap)

½ small wholemeal scone (25 g)

3 Ryvitas or 4 rye Cruskits

4 x 9 Grains Vita-Weats

1 UNIT LEGUMES

160 g cooked, drained lentils

80 g cooked, drained chickpeas or red kidney beans

100 g cooked, drained cannellini beans or four-bean mix

1 UNIT LOW-GI, HIGH-STARCH VEGETABLES

100 g sweet potato

70 g corn

100 g green peas or broad beans

200 g pumpkin

1 UNIT GRAINS

15 g wholemeal plain or self-raising flour, cornflour, rice flour, arrowroot or green banana flour

⅓ cup cooked rice

20 g raw (40 g cooked) quinoa or couscous

Dairy

3 units per day

Choose from:

1 UNIT DAIRY

150 ml milk or 200 ml skim milk or low-fat calcium-enriched soy or almond milk

80 g natural Greek-style yoghurt or 100 g low-fat natural Greek-style yoghurt or low-fat, lactose-free soy yoghurt

20 g cheddar, parmesan, Swiss or feta cheese

55 g ricotta or cottage cheese

25 g mozzarella or bocconcini cheese, or low-fat cream cheese

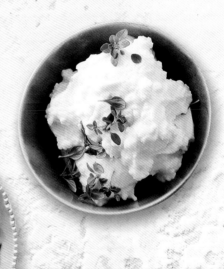

YOUR DAILY FOOD GUIDE FOR LEVEL 1 (6000 kJ)

Lean meat, fish, poultry, eggs, tofu

2.5 units per day

For lunch, choose from:

1 UNIT LEAN MEAT, FISH, POULTRY, EGGS, TOFU
100 g (cooked weight) lean meat or fish: chicken, turkey, pork, beef, lamb or tinned or fresh fish or seafood
2 small eggs (40–42 g/½ unit each)
100 g tofu
We recommend fish for lunch at least twice a week.

> If you wish to have an egg for breakfast, just have 50 g less meat at lunchtime to account for this.

For dinner, choose from:

1.5 UNITS LEAN MEAT, FISH, POULTRY, EGGS, TOFU
150 g (raw weight) lean meat or fish: chicken, turkey, pork, beef, lamb, fish or seafood
3 eggs (50 g/½ unit each)
150 g tofu
We recommend fish for dinner at least twice a week and red meat no more than three times a week.

> You may not wish to eat red meat, fish or chicken — or not every day. Legumes are an excellent source of protein for vegetarians or vegans, although they are higher in carbohydrates than their animal-based counterparts, so keep this in mind when planning your daily intake.
> 1 unit of legumes is as follows:
>
> - 160 g cooked, drained lentils (provides 15 g carbs and 11 g protein)
> - 80 g cooked, drained chickpeas or red kidney beans (provides 12 g carbs and 6 g protein)
> - 100 g cooked, drained cannellini beans or four-bean mix (provides 13 g carbs and 6 g protein).

Low–moderate carbohydrate vegetables

At least 5 units per day

Choose from:

1 UNIT LOW-CARBOHYDRATE VEGETABLES
(AT LEAST 3 UNITS OF THESE PER DAY)
½ cup (75 g) cooked vegetables
1 cup (150 g) salad vegetables

Low-carbohydrate vegetables: *lettuce, broccoli, broccolini, spinach, artichoke (high in resistant starch), bok choy, asparagus, bean sprouts, cucumber, mushrooms, tomato, zucchini, kale, rocket, garlic, chilli, fresh herbs and spices.*

1 UNIT MODERATE-CARBOHYDRATE VEGETABLES
(UP TO 2 UNITS PER DAY)
½ cup (75 g) cooked vegetables
1 cup (150 g) salad vegetables

Moderate-carbohydrate vegetables: *cauliflower, celery, green beans, capsicum (all colours), brussels sprouts, cabbage, spring onion, snow peas, carrot, eggplant, onion, leek, parsnip, swede, bamboo shoots, fennel, turnip and radish.*

> Strawberries are a very low-carb fruit and can be substituted for a moderate-carb vegetable if you wish (100 g = 1 unit).

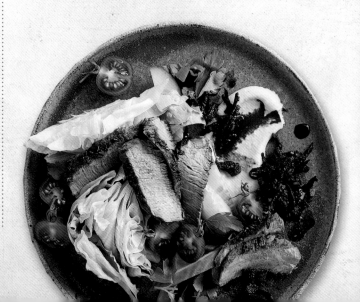

Healthy fats

10 units a day

Choose from:

1 UNIT HEALTHY FATS

5 g (1 teaspoon) olive, grapeseed or sunflower oil

5 g (1 teaspoon) tahini (sesame butter)

20 g avocado

20 g (1 tablespoon) hummus

5 g (1 teaspoon) olive oil, canola or Nuttelex margarine

10 g nuts (almonds, cashews, pecans or walnuts)

> **Nuts are a primary source of healthy fats in the Low-carb Diet. We encourage you to eat at least 60 g (6 units) of nuts each day.**

Indulgence foods

2 units per week

Choose from:

1 UNIT INDULGENCE FOOD

Any food or drink providing approximately 450 kJ — e.g. 150 ml wine, 20 g chocolate, 40 g store-bought low-fat dips, 10 Arnotts Shapes, 1 x 20 g packet of chips, 10 Pringles, ½ slice of pizza or 35 g hot chips.

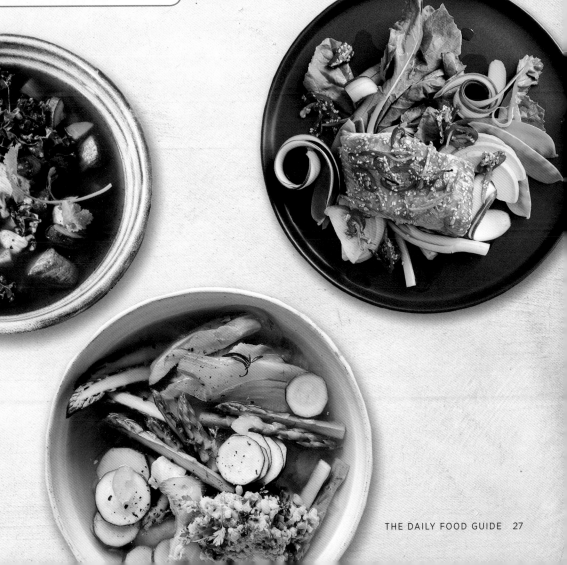

HOW TO BUILD A DAILY MEAL PLAN

Once you have determined your level from page 21, write down your daily allowance and pop it on the fridge or in your diary, and you'll always have this information on hand to refer to. If you move between levels at any point, be sure to update this accordingly. For example, if you are on level 1 (6000 kJ), this is what your daily allowance will look like:

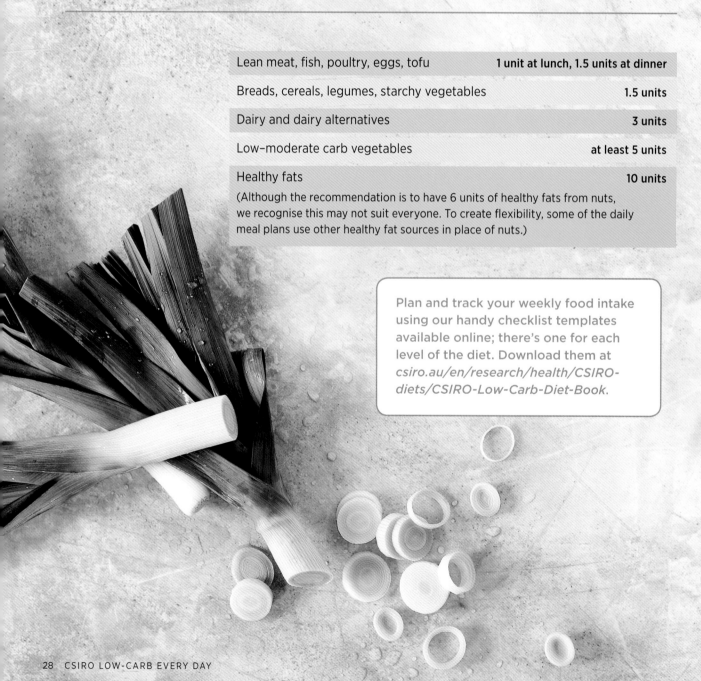

Lean meat, fish, poultry, eggs, tofu	**1 unit at lunch, 1.5 units at dinner**
Breads, cereals, legumes, starchy vegetables	**1.5 units**
Dairy and dairy alternatives	**3 units**
Low–moderate carb vegetables	**at least 5 units**
Healthy fats	**10 units**

(Although the recommendation is to have 6 units of healthy fats from nuts, we recognise this may not suit everyone. To create flexibility, some of the daily meal plans use other healthy fat sources in place of nuts.)

> Plan and track your weekly food intake using our handy checklist templates available online; there's one for each level of the diet. Download them at *csiro.au/en/research/health/CSIRO-diets/CSIRO-Low-Carb-Diet-Book*.

You can choose from the recipes and/or the meal builders to construct a daily meal plan that fits your daily allowance. Below is an example of just one way you could do this...

1

Choose a lunch and dinner option from the recipe section and note their unit value:

LUNCH

TUNA, CHEESE AND VEGETABLE SLICE
Lean meat, fish, poultry, eggs, tofu: 1
Breads, cereals, legumes, starchy vegetables: 0.5
Dairy and dairy alternatives: 1
Low–moderate carb vegetables: 2.5
Healthy fats: 2

DINNER

LEMON AND GARLIC CHICKEN STEW
Lean meat, fish, poultry, eggs, tofu: 1.5
Low–moderate carb vegetables: 3
Healthy fats: 2

2

Use the suggestions on the meal builder pages to put together a breakfast option, then determine your portion sizes using the information on the daily food guide:

BREAKFAST MEAL BUILDER 3
- raw (natural) oats (30 g for 1 bread/cereal unit)
- calcium-enriched almond milk (200 ml for 1 dairy unit)
- toasted mixed nuts (30 g for 3 healthy fat units)
- mixed spice (free)

3

Then add a snack to round out the units for the day:

SNACK
30 g nuts (3 healthy fat units)

Alternatively, look at the daily plans we have put together for you on the following pages.

DAILY MEAL PLAN 1: EGGS FOR BREAKFAST

Many people love having eggs for breakfast, so to enable them to do that on the diet we have devised a day plan that incorporates these units spread across the day.

BREAKFAST

2 small fried eggs (½ unit lean meat, fish etc) + **3 asparagus spears** (1 unit low–mod veg) + **1 tbsp ricotta** (½ unit dairy) + **1 teaspoon olive oil** (1 unit healthy fats) + **½ piece mountain bread** (1 unit bread/cereal) + **fennel seeds**

LUNCH

Herb Chicken Patties with Supergreen Lentil Salad, page 64 (1 unit lean meat, fish etc + 3 units low–mod veg + 1 unit dairy + 2 units healthy fats + ½ unit bread/cereal)

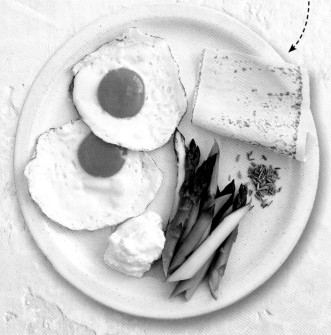

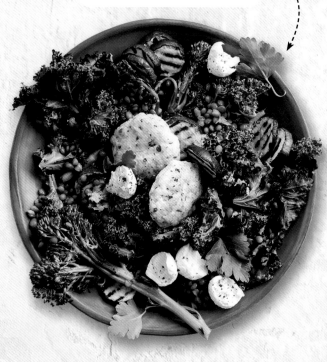

DINNER

Zucchini and Ricotta Pie with Avocado and Pecan Salad, page 152 (1 unit lean meat, fish etc + 3 units low–mod veg + 1 unit dairy + 4 units healthy fats)

SNACK

30 g almonds (2 units healthy fat) + **cup of coffee** + **75 ml milk** (½ unit dairy)

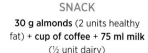

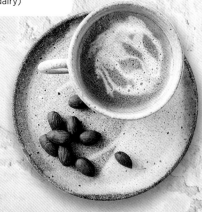

Together these meals make up your daily units and carb allowance for level 1 (6000 kJ)

Keeping your pantry well-stocked with these items means you will always have what you need to create delicious homecooked meals.

almonds (raw, ground, blanched)
macadamias
mixed nuts and seeds (toasted)
mini wholemeal pita bread
mountain bread
pistachios (unsalted shelled)
pecans
pine nuts
pure vanilla extract
raw (natural) oats
Ryvita crispbread
salt-reduced chicken stock
salt-reduced vegetable stock
tahini

tinned cannellini beans
tinned lentils
tinned tuna in springwater

SAUCES & CONDIMENTS
olive oil spray
extra virgin olive oil
sesame oil
wholegrain mustard
Shaoxing rice wine or dry sherry
balsamic vinegar
red wine vinegar
white wine vinegar
oyster sauce
rice bran oil

HERBS & SPICES
Chinese five spice
fennel seeds
ground ginger
ground turmeric
mixed spice
dried mixed herbs
garlic powder
smoked paprika

FRIDGE
garlic
ginger
eggs
milk

low-fat natural Greek-style yoghurt
ricotta
cottage cheese
cheddar
feta
silken tofu
firm tofu

FREEZER
frozen peas
frozen shelled edamame

SHOPPING LIST

QUANTITY	ITEM
. . . .	**asparagus spears**
. . . .	**avocado**
. . . .	**broccolini**
. . . .	**cherry bocconcini**
. . . .	**lean chicken tenderloins**
. . . .	**chives**
. . . .	**tarragon**
. . . .	**flat-leaf parsley**
. . . .	**kale leaves**
. . . .	**lemons**
. . . .	**thyme**
. . . .	**yellow and green zucchini**

Or try these alternatives

LUNCH (give the meal builders a go):
- 100 g tinned tuna + 1 cup mixed salad leaves + 1 cup artichoke hearts in brine + 50 g lentils + 40 g avocado + 55 g ricotta + French dressing (page 56) and herb topper (page 52)
- 100 g chicken tenderloin + 1 cup baby spinach leaves + 1 cup chopped zucchini + 50 g cannellini beans + 20 g toasted pecans + 40 g bocconcini + Italian dressing (page 56) and herb topper (page 52)

DINNER (choose one of the following):
- One-pan Chilli-soy Salmon (page 95)
- Beetroot and Beef Rissoles with Herb Salad and Mustard Tahini (page 129)

DAILY MEAL PLAN 2: A LIGHT LUNCH

If you like a smaller meal in the middle of the day, here's
a way for you to build up your units as the day progresses.

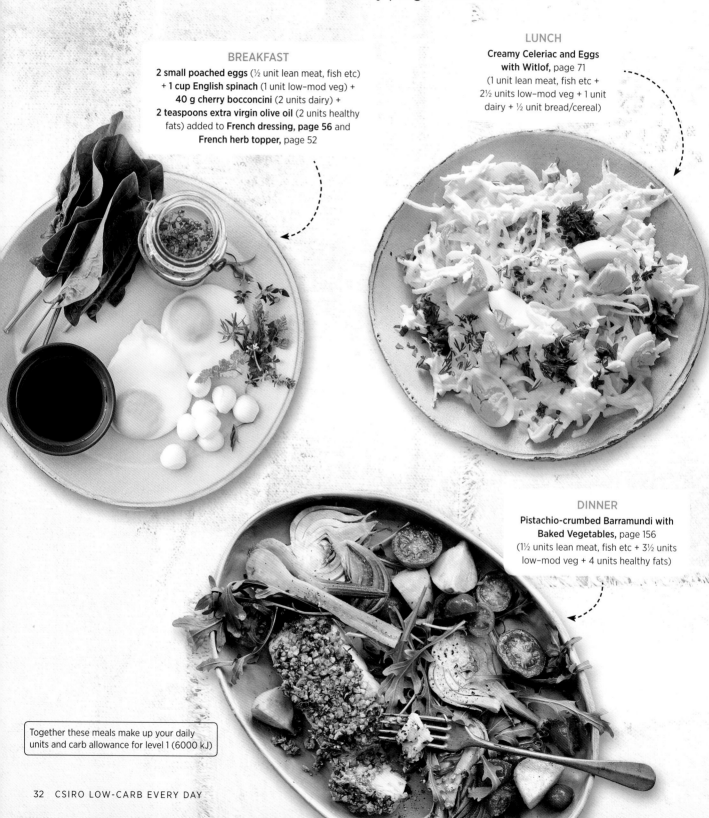

BREAKFAST

2 small poached eggs (½ unit lean meat, fish etc)
+ **1 cup English spinach** (1 unit low–mod veg) +
40 g cherry bocconcini (2 units dairy) +
2 teaspoons extra virgin olive oil (2 units healthy
fats) added to **French dressing, page 56** and
French herb topper, page 52

LUNCH

**Creamy Celeriac and Eggs
with Witlof,** page 71
(1 unit lean meat, fish etc +
2½ units low–mod veg + 1 unit
dairy + ½ unit bread/cereal)

DINNER

**Pistachio-crumbed Barramundi with
Baked Vegetables,** page 156
(1½ units lean meat, fish etc + 3½ units
low–mod veg + 4 units healthy fats)

Together these meals make up your daily
units and carb allowance for level 1 (6000 kJ)

SHOPPING LIST

QUANTITY	ITEM
. . . .	avocado
. . . .	baby fennel
. . . .	baby rocket leaves
. . . .	barramundi fillets
. . . .	celeriac
. . . .	cherry bocconcini
. . . .	cherry tomatoes
. . . .	chervil
. . . .	chives
. . . .	English spinach
. . . .	tarragon
. . . .	lemon
. . . .	oregano
. . . .	red onion
. . . .	rosemary
. . . .	thyme
. . . .	small yellow squash
. . . .	green witlof
. . . .	zucchini

SNACK

1 Ryvita crispbread (½ unit bread/cereal)
+ **40 g avocado** (2 units healthy fats) +
10 g tahini (2 units healthy fats) + **cherry
tomatoes** (½ unit low–mod veg)

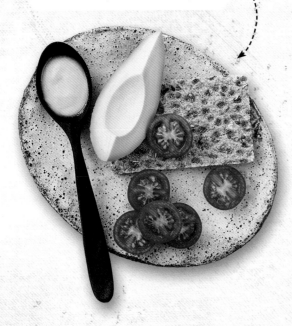

Or try these alternatives

LUNCH (choose one of the following):

- Tofu and Edamame San Choy Bau (page 82) + snack of 50 g low-fat natural Greek-style yoghurt
- Ginger Cashew Chicken with Edamame Zucchini Noodles (page 76) + 1 small latte or cappuccino (no sugar)

DINNER (choose one of the following):

- Beef Fillet with Mushroom Salad and Homemade Barbecue Sauce (page 141) + 200 g low-fat natural Greek-style yoghurt
  + 20 g flaked almonds and cinnamon
- Roast Chicken with Whipped Ricotta (page 160) + 20 g smashed avocado

DAILY MEAL PLAN 3: SPECIAL WEEKENDS

We all like to eat special meals on the weekends, especially if friends are coming over. Here is an eating plan that will keep you nourished and satisfied without feeling like you're missing out on anything.

BREAKFAST

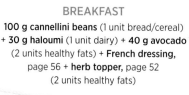

100 g cannellini beans (1 unit bread/cereal) + **30 g haloumi** (1 unit dairy) + **40 g avocado** (2 units healthy fats) + **French dressing**, page 56 + **herb topper**, page 52 (2 units healthy fats)

LUNCH

Herb Chicken Patties with Supergreen Lentil Salad, page 64 (1 unit lean meat, fish etc + 3 units low–mod veg + 1 unit dairy + 2 units healthy fats + ½ unit bread/cereal)

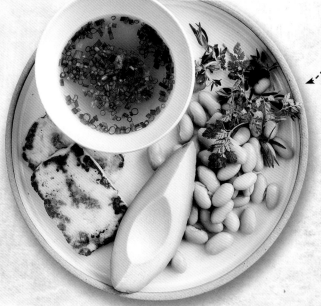

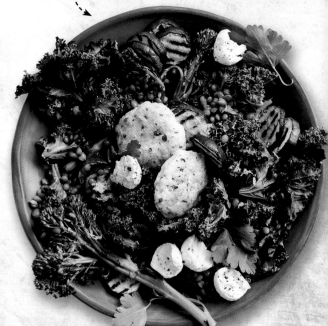

DINNER

Thai Chicken and Supergreens Curry, page 170 (1½ units lean meat, fish etc + 3 units low–mod veg + 3 units healthy fats) + **100 g low-fat natural Greek-style yoghurt** (1 unit dairy; yoghurt not shown)

Together these meals make up your daily units and carb allowance for level 1 (6000 kJ)

SHOPPING LIST

QUANTITY	ITEM		QUANTITY	ITEM
. . . .	avocado		. . . .	flat-leaf parsley
. . . .	baby spinach leaves		. . . .	tarragon
. . . .	bean sprouts		. . . .	haloumi
. . . .	Chinese broccoli		. . . .	kaffir lime leaves
. . . .	broccolini		. . . .	kale
. . . .	cherry bocconcini		. . . .	lemon
. . . .	chervil		. . . .	lemongrass
. . . .	long green chillies (fresh)		. . . .	lime
. . . .	green beans		. . . .	spring onions
. . . .	lean chicken breast fillets		. . . .	sugar snap peas
. . . .	lean chicken tenderloins		. . . .	thyme
. . . .	chives		. . . .	zucchini
. . . .	coriander			

SNACK

60 g avocado (3 units healthy fats; can be added to salad at lunch if desired)

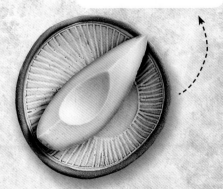

Or try these alternatives

LUNCH (choose one of the following):
- Chicken with Creamy Celeriac Slaw (page 79)
- Zucchini and Ricotta Pie with Avocado and Pecan Salad (page 152) + 1 crispbread + 20 g extra avocado

DINNER (choose one of the following):
- Lamb and Vegetable Massaman Curry (page 166) + 200 g low-fat natural Greek-style yoghurt
- Beef and Vegetable Lasagne (page 162) + 1½ cups packed greens

DAILY MEAL PLAN 4: MEALS ON-THE-GO

If you're on the move all day, you shouldn't feel like you need to sacrifice healthy eating. These meals can be prepped and packed in advance, and fulfil all your nutritional needs. You won't have to resort to processed foods with these on board!

BREAKFAST

30 g raw (natural) oats (1 unit bread/cereal) + **200 ml almond milk** (1 unit dairy) + **20 g toasted mixed nuts and seeds** (2 units healthy fats) + mixed spice

LUNCH

Tuna, Cheese and Vegetable Slice, page 63 (1 unit lean meat, fish etc + 2½ units low–mod veg + 1 unit dairy + 2 units healthy fats + ½ unit bread/cereal) + **2 cups salad greens** (2 units low–mod veg)

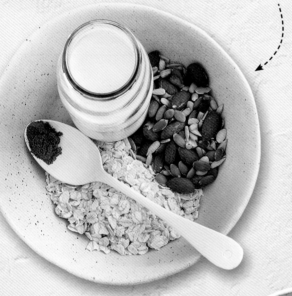

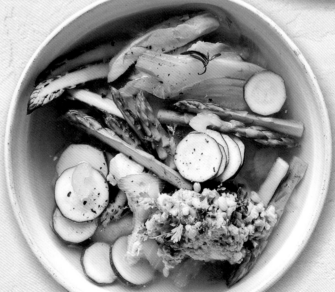

DINNER

Spring Chicken Stew with Zesty Avocado, page 206 (1½ units lean meat, fish etc + 4 units low–mod veg + 3 units healthy fats)

Together these meals make up your daily units and carb allowance for level 1 (6000 kJ)

SHOPPING LIST

QUANTITY	ITEM
. . . .	almond milk
. . . .	asparagus
. . . .	avocado
. . . .	baby fennel
. . . .	small basil leaves
. . . .	broccoli
. . . .	celery
. . . .	lean chicken tenderloins
. . . .	chervil

QUANTITY	ITEM
. . . .	cucumber
. . . .	Lebanese cucumber
. . . .	tarragon
. . . .	iceberg lettuce
. . . .	lemon thyme
. . . .	limes
. . . .	mixed berries
. . . .	zucchini

SNACK

50 g mixed berries + cucumber sticks (1 unit low–mod veg) + **55 g ricotta** (1 unit dairy) + **20 g almonds** (2 units healthy fats)

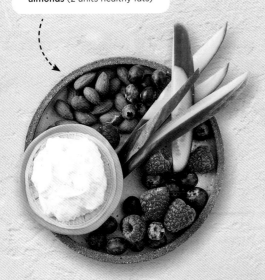

Or try these alternatives

LUNCH (choose one of the following):
- Vegetable Stuffed Egg Rolls with Macadamia Parsley Dukkah (page 80)

DINNER (choose one of the following):
- Tuna and Zucchini Bake with Lemony Greens (page 193)
- Chicken, Silverbeet and Lentil Dhal (page 194)

DAILY MEAL PLAN 5: **VEGETARIAN**

Whether you are vegetarian or just like to eat meat-free now and then, this daily plan will tick all the boxes. It also includes a serve of carbohydrate extra as the optional snack.

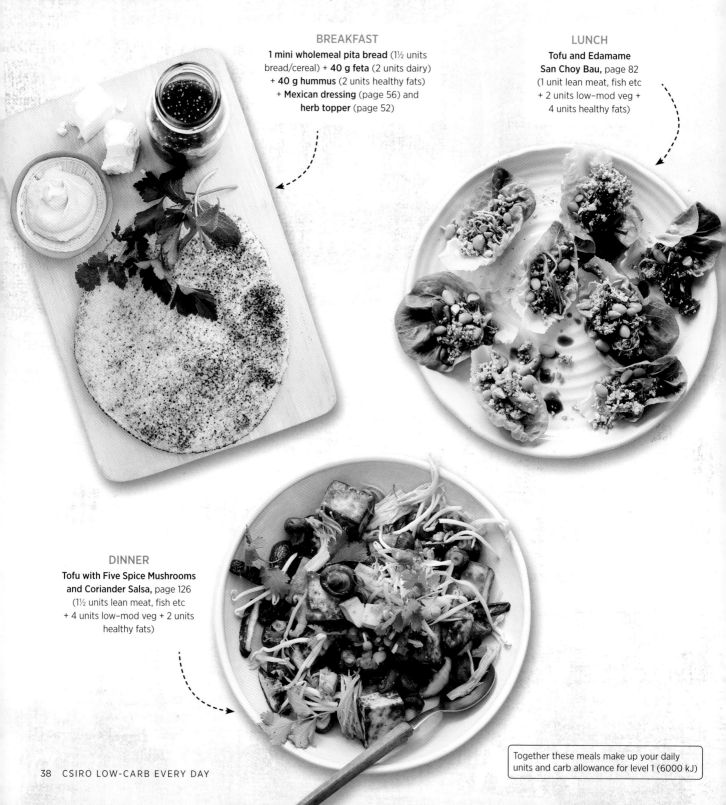

BREAKFAST
1 mini wholemeal pita bread (1½ units bread/cereal) + **40 g feta** (2 units dairy) + **40 g hummus** (2 units healthy fats) + **Mexican dressing** (page 56) and **herb topper** (page 52)

LUNCH
Tofu and Edamame San Choy Bau, page 82 (1 unit lean meat, fish etc + 2 units low–mod veg + 4 units healthy fats)

DINNER
Tofu with Five Spice Mushrooms and Coriander Salsa, page 126 (1½ units lean meat, fish etc + 4 units low–mod veg + 2 units healthy fats)

Together these meals make up your daily units and carb allowance for level 1 (6000 kJ)

SHOPPING LIST

QUANTITY	ITEM
. . . .	avocado
. . . .	baby cos lettuce
. . . .	bean sprouts
. . . .	fresh long red chilli
. . . .	chives
. . . .	coriander
. . . .	flat-leaf parsley
. . . .	green beans

QUANTITY	ITEM
. . . .	hummus
. . . .	limes
. . . .	mint
. . . .	mixed mushrooms
. . . .	spring onions
. . . .	strawberries

SNACK
1 serve of **Strawberries with Ginger Ricotta,** page 215
(1 unit dairy + 2 units healthy fats + 1 carbohydrate extra)

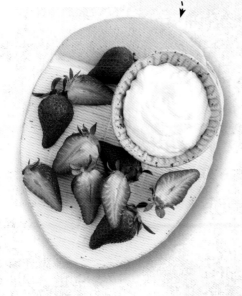

Or try these alternatives

LUNCH (choose one of the following):
- Cheesy Asparagus and Broccoli Frittata (page 81; made with 2 teaspoons rice bran oil instead of oil spray)
- Zucchini and Ricotta Pie with Avocado and Pecan Salad (page 152) + 1 wholegrain crispbread topped with sliced cucumber

DINNER (choose one of the following):
- Pesto Tofu with Raw Vegetable Noodles (page 111)
- Tofu Falafel Fritters with Braised Greens (page 151)

BREAKFAST MEAL BUILDERS

Six great breakfast ideas, from top to bottom

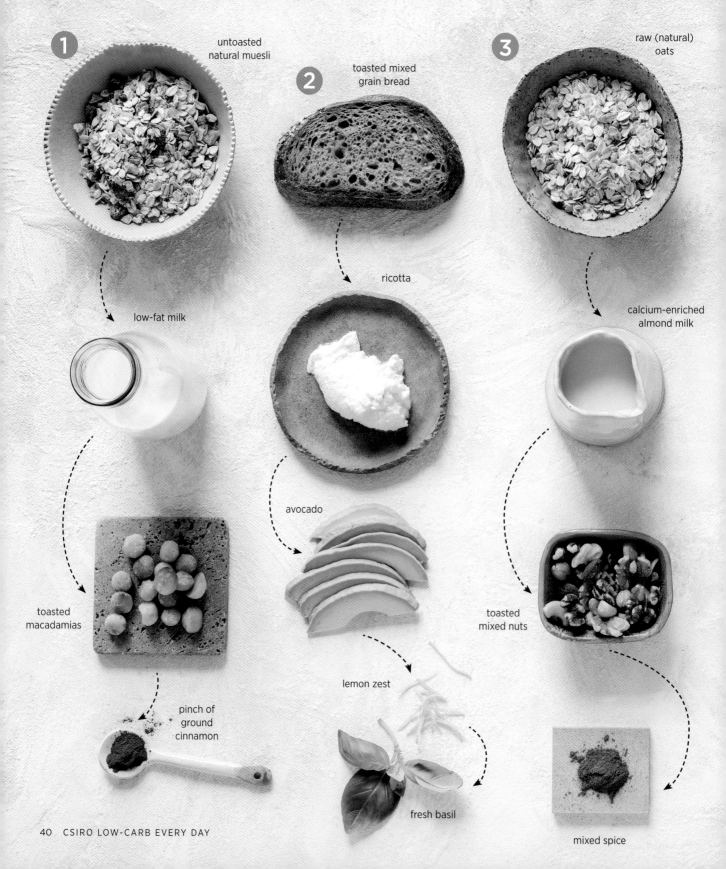

1 untoasted natural muesli

2 toasted mixed grain bread

3 raw (natural) oats

ricotta

low-fat milk

calcium-enriched almond milk

avocado

toasted macadamias

toasted mixed nuts

lemon zest

pinch of ground cinnamon

fresh basil

mixed spice

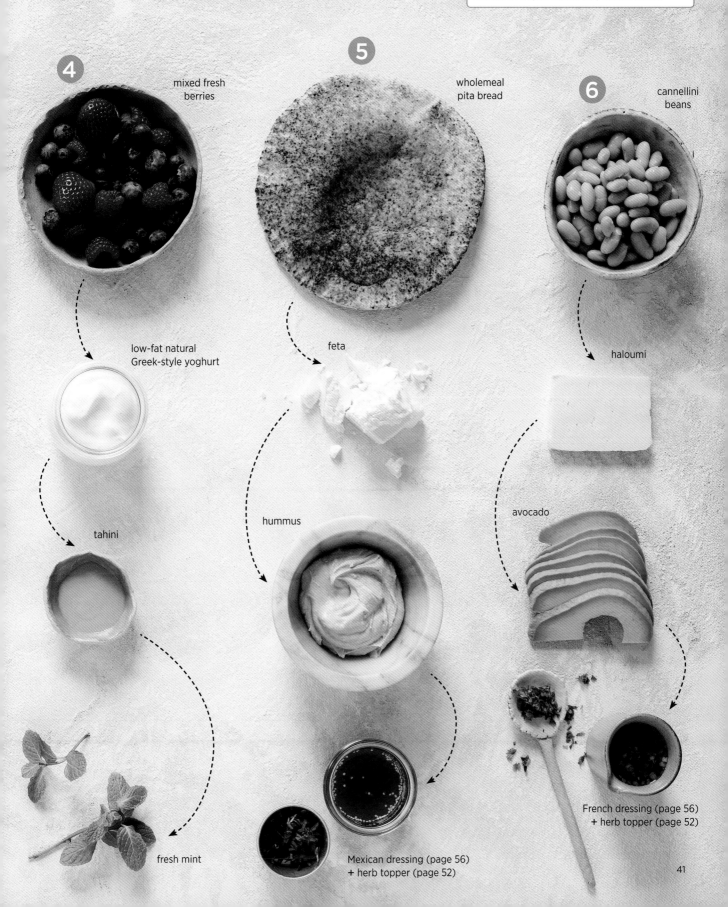

Portions shown here are a guide only. Use the daily food guide (see pages 25–27) to determine portion size based on your overall daily unit allowance.

4

mixed fresh berries

5

wholemeal pita bread

6

cannellini beans

low-fat natural Greek-style yoghurt

feta

haloumi

tahini

hummus

avocado

fresh mint

Mexican dressing (page 56) + herb topper (page 52)

French dressing (page 56) + herb topper (page 52)

41

EGG MEAL BUILDERS

Love eggs? Here are four delicious options, from left to right

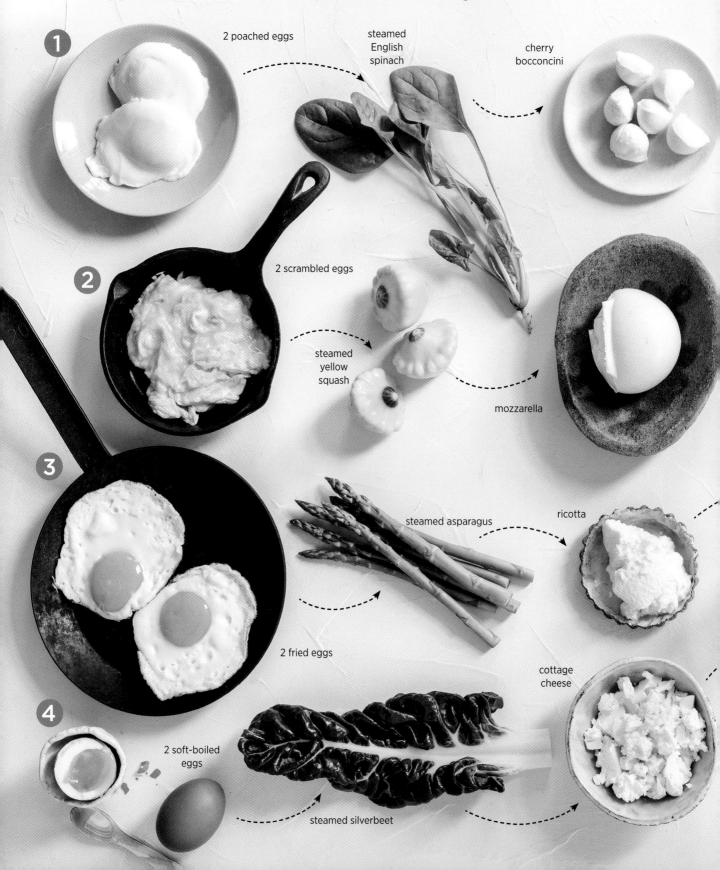

1 2 poached eggs · steamed English spinach · cherry bocconcini

2 2 scrambled eggs · steamed yellow squash · mozzarella

3 2 fried eggs · steamed asparagus · ricotta

4 2 soft-boiled eggs · steamed silverbeet · cottage cheese

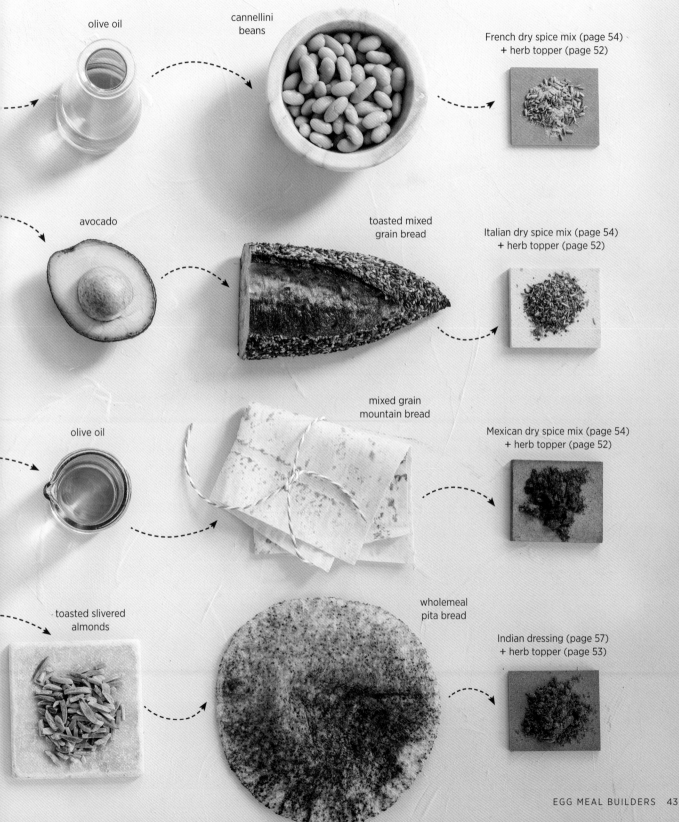

Portions shown here are a guide only. Use the daily food guide (see pages 25–27) to determine portion size based on your overall daily unit allowance.

olive oil

cannellini beans

French dry spice mix (page 54) + herb topper (page 52)

avocado

toasted mixed grain bread

Italian dry spice mix (page 54) + herb topper (page 52)

olive oil

mixed grain mountain bread

Mexican dry spice mix (page 54) + herb topper (page 52)

toasted slivered almonds

wholemeal pita bread

Indian dressing (page 57) + herb topper (page 53)

PORTABLE SALAD MEAL BUILDERS

Four sensational salads, from left to right

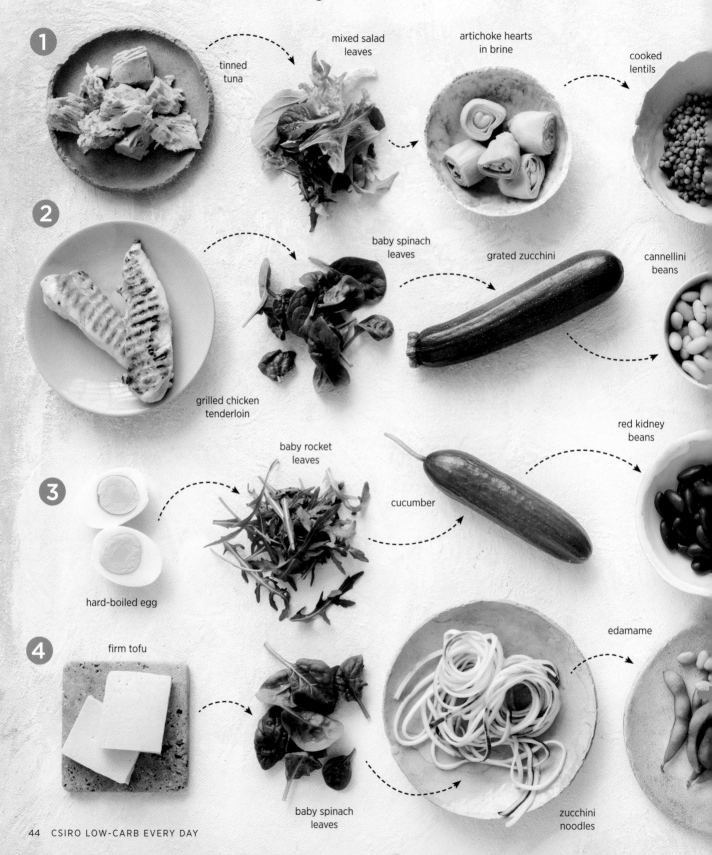

1 tinned tuna → mixed salad leaves → artichoke hearts in brine → cooked lentils

2 grilled chicken tenderloin → baby spinach leaves → grated zucchini → cannellini beans

3 hard-boiled egg → baby rocket leaves → cucumber → red kidney beans

4 firm tofu → baby spinach leaves → zucchini noodles → edamame

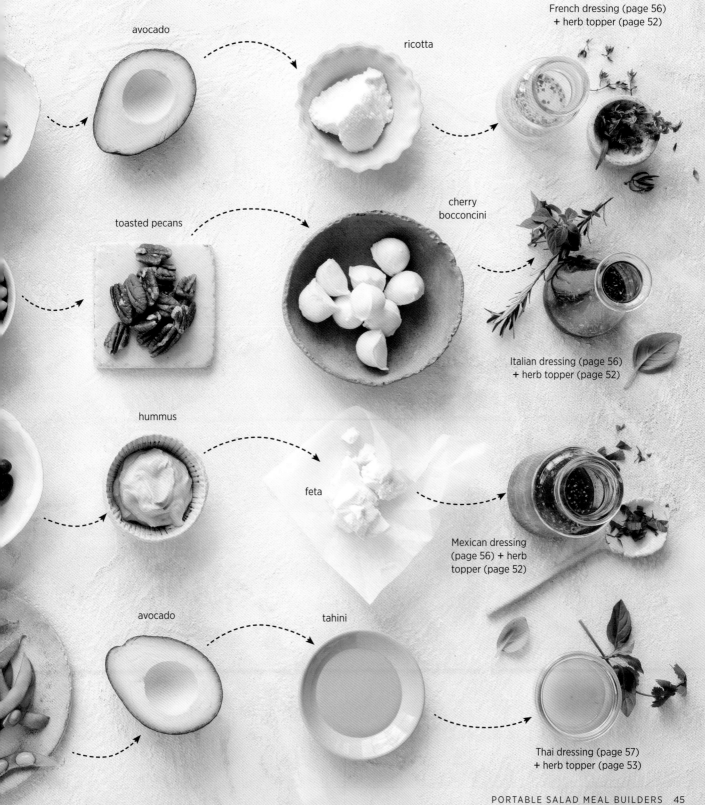

Portions shown here are a guide only. Use the daily food guide (see pages 25–27) to determine portion size based on your overall daily unit allowance.

avocado

ricotta

French dressing (page 56) + herb topper (page 52)

toasted pecans

cherry bocconcini

Italian dressing (page 56) + herb topper (page 52)

hummus

feta

Mexican dressing (page 56) + herb topper (page 52)

avocado

tahini

Thai dressing (page 57) + herb topper (page 53)

CRISPBREAD TOPPER MEAL BUILDERS

The possibilities are endless! Here are six tasty options, from left to right

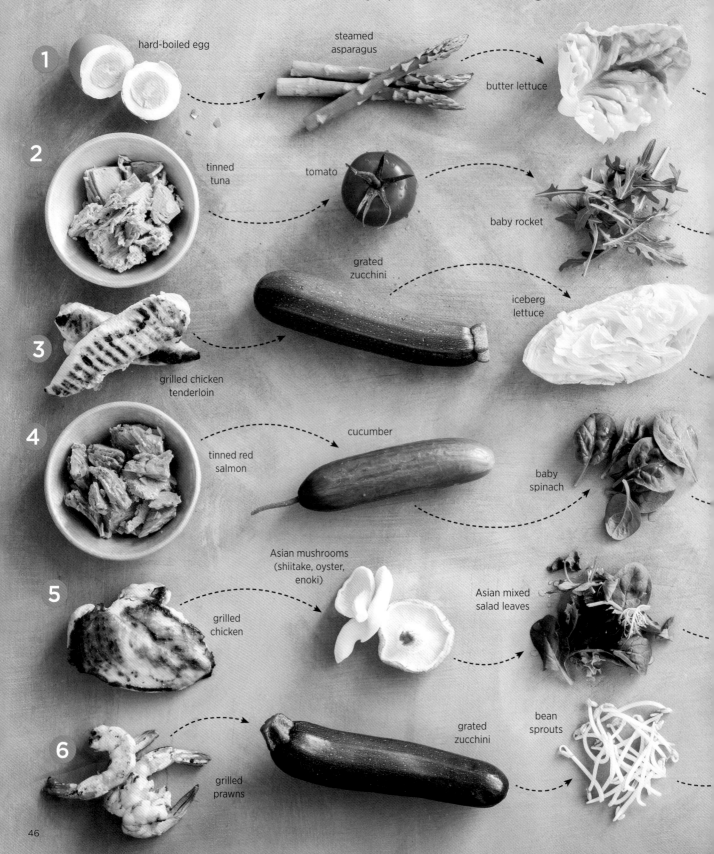

1 hard-boiled egg → steamed asparagus → butter lettuce

2 tinned tuna → tomato → baby rocket

3 grilled chicken tenderloin → grated zucchini → iceberg lettuce

4 tinned red salmon → cucumber → baby spinach

5 grilled chicken → Asian mushrooms (shiitake, oyster, enoki) → Asian mixed salad leaves

6 grilled prawns → grated zucchini → bean sprouts

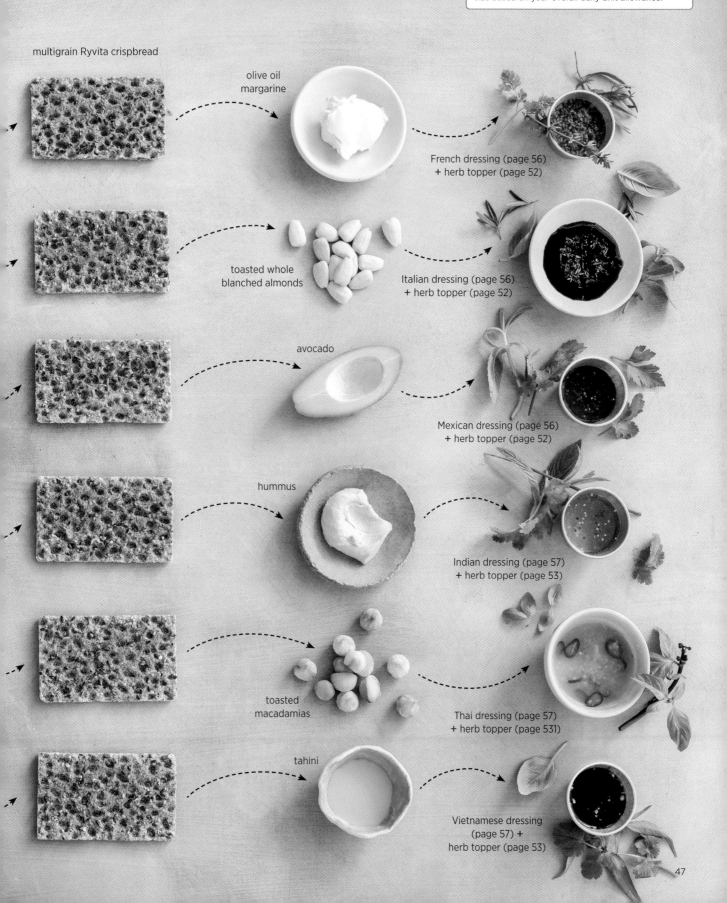

Portions shown here are a guide only. Use the daily food guide (see pages 25–27) to determine portion size based on your overall daily unit allowance.

multigrain Ryvita crispbread

olive oil margarine

French dressing (page 56)
+ herb topper (page 52)

toasted whole blanched almonds

Italian dressing (page 56)
+ herb topper (page 52)

avocado

Mexican dressing (page 56)
+ herb topper (page 52)

hummus

Indian dressing (page 57)
+ herb topper (page 53)

toasted macadamias

Thai dressing (page 57)
+ herb topper (page 531)

tahini

Vietnamese dressing
(page 57) +
herb topper (page 53)

CHICKEN MEAL BUILDERS

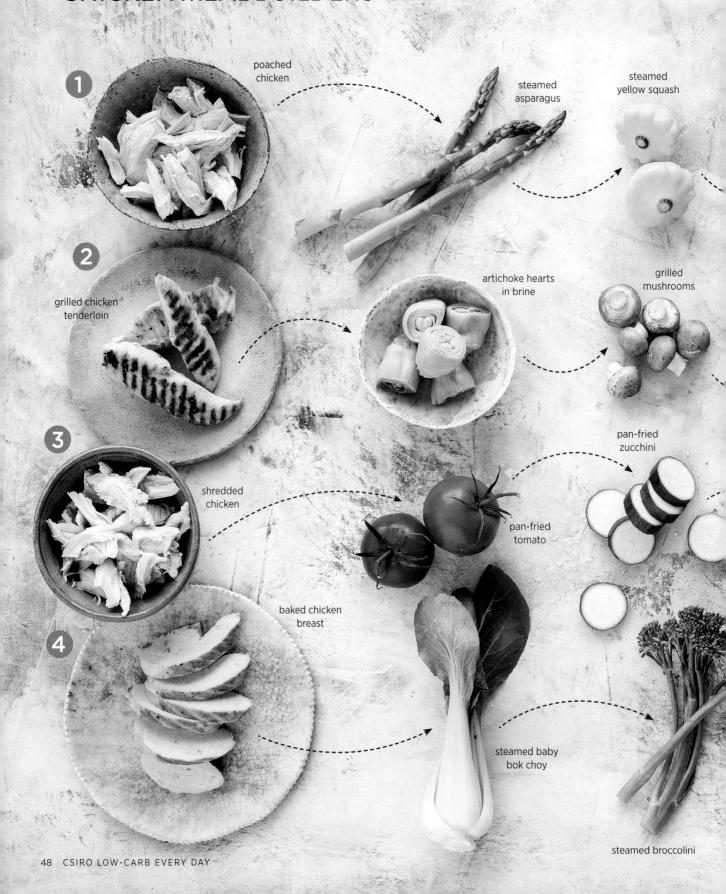

1 poached chicken

steamed asparagus

steamed yellow squash

2 grilled chicken tenderloin

artichoke hearts in brine

grilled mushrooms

3 shredded chicken

pan-fried zucchini

pan-fried tomato

4 baked chicken breast

steamed baby bok choy

steamed broccolini

Portions shown here are a guide only. Use the daily food guide (see pages 25–27) to determine portion size based on your overall daily unit allowance.

steamed fennel
avocado + feta
French dry spice mix (page 54) + dressing (page 56) + herb topper (page 52)
grilled eggplant
tahini + cherry bocconcini
Italian dry spice mix (page 54) + dressing (page 56) + herb topper (page 52)
pan-fried capsicum
hummus
Mexican dry spice mix (page 54) + dressing (page 56) + herb topper (page 52)
steamed snow peas
avocado
Thai dry spice mix (page 55) + dressing (page 57) + herb topper (page 53)

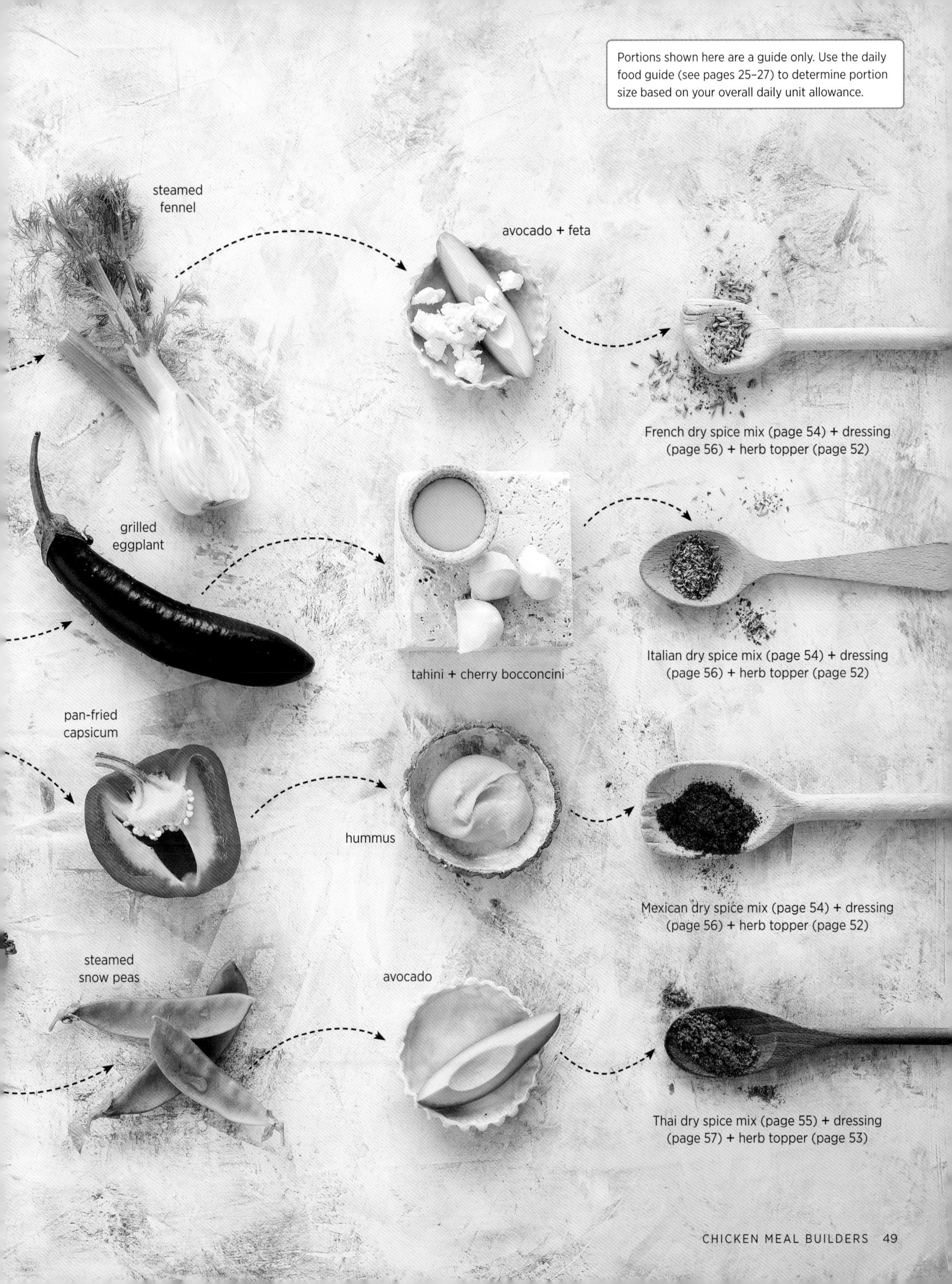

MEAT & SEAFOOD MEAL BUILDERS

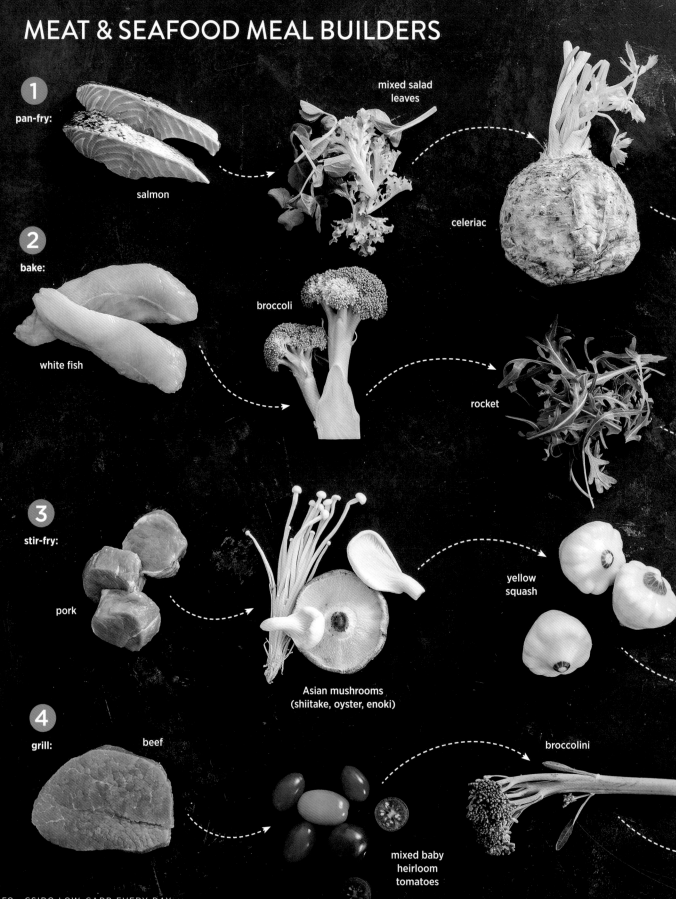

1 pan-fry: salmon

mixed salad leaves

celeriac

2 bake: white fish

broccoli

rocket

3 stir-fry: pork

Asian mushrooms (shiitake, oyster, enoki)

yellow squash

4 grill: beef

mixed baby heirloom tomatoes

broccolini

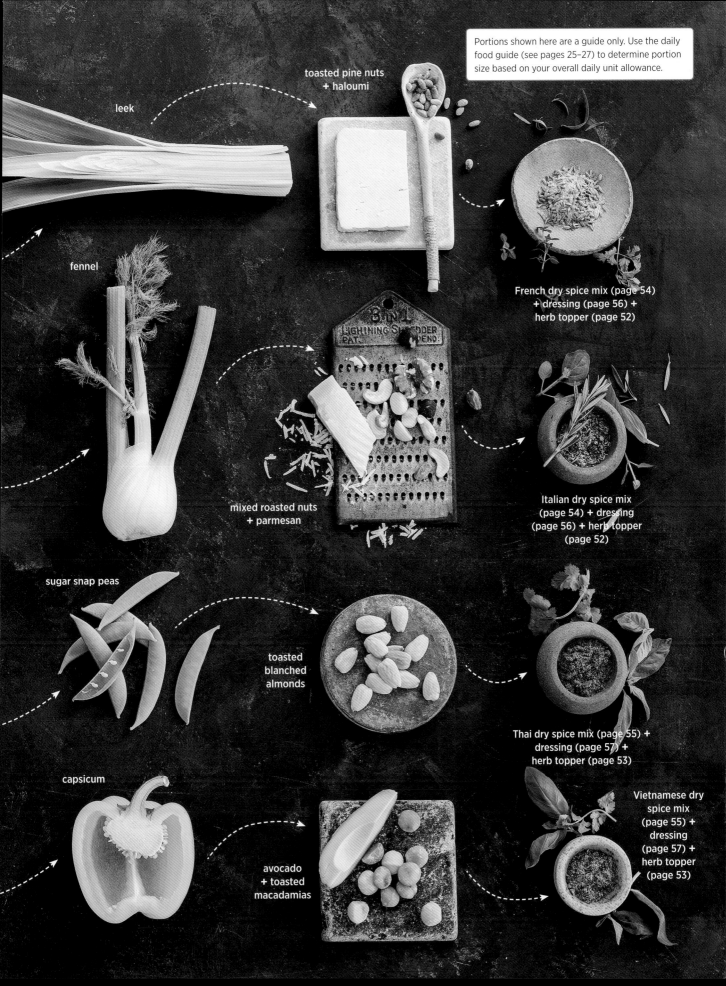

leek

toasted pine nuts
+ haloumi

Portions shown here are a guide only. Use the daily food guide (see pages 25–27) to determine portion size based on your overall daily unit allowance.

French dry spice mix (page 54)
+ dressing (page 56) +
herb topper (page 52)

fennel

mixed roasted nuts
+ parmesan

Italian dry spice mix
(page 54) + dressing
(page 56) + herb topper
(page 52)

sugar snap peas

toasted
blanched
almonds

Thai dry spice mix (page 55) +
dressing (page 57) +
herb topper (page 53)

capsicum

Vietnamese dry
spice mix
(page 55) +
dressing
(page 57) +
herb topper
(page 53)

avocado
+ toasted
macadamias

FLAVOUR BOOSTERS: HERB TOPPERS

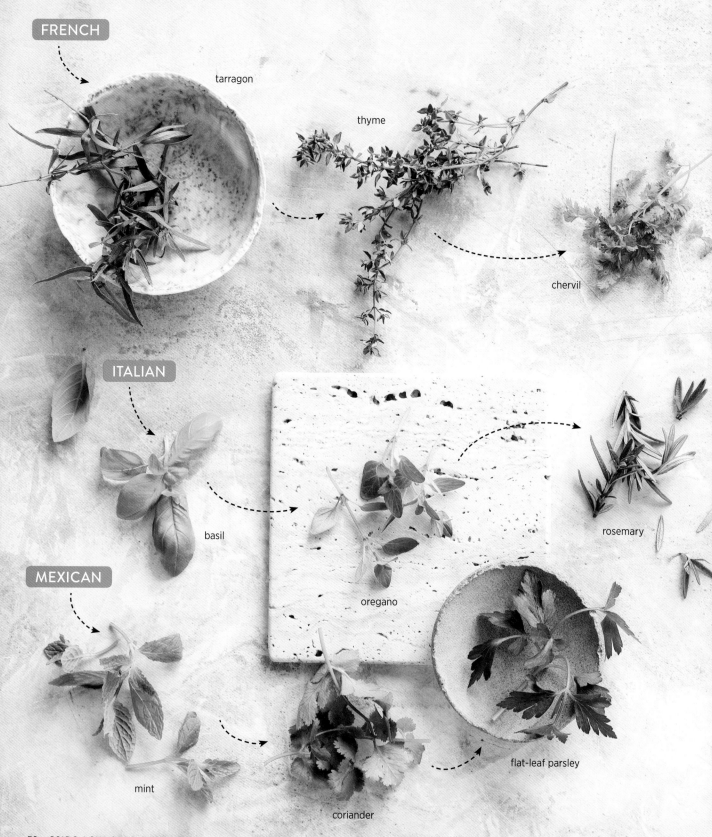

FRENCH

tarragon

thyme

chervil

ITALIAN

basil

oregano

rosemary

MEXICAN

mint

coriander

flat-leaf parsley

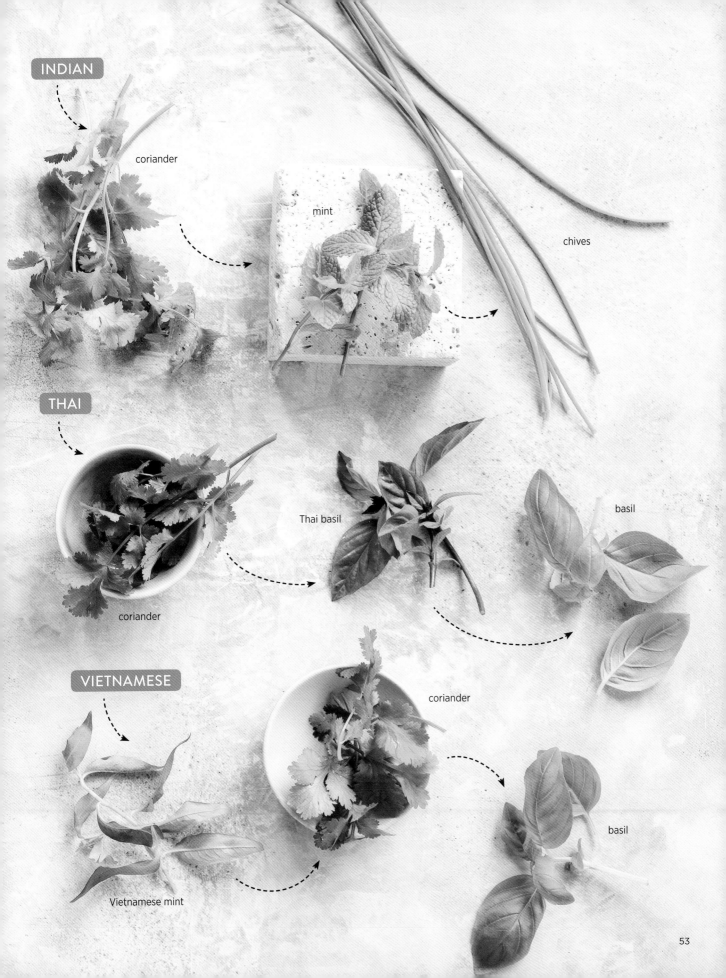

INDIAN

coriander

mint

chives

THAI

coriander

Thai basil

basil

VIETNAMESE

coriander

Vietnamese mint

basil

53

FLAVOUR BOOSTERS: DRY SPICE MIXES

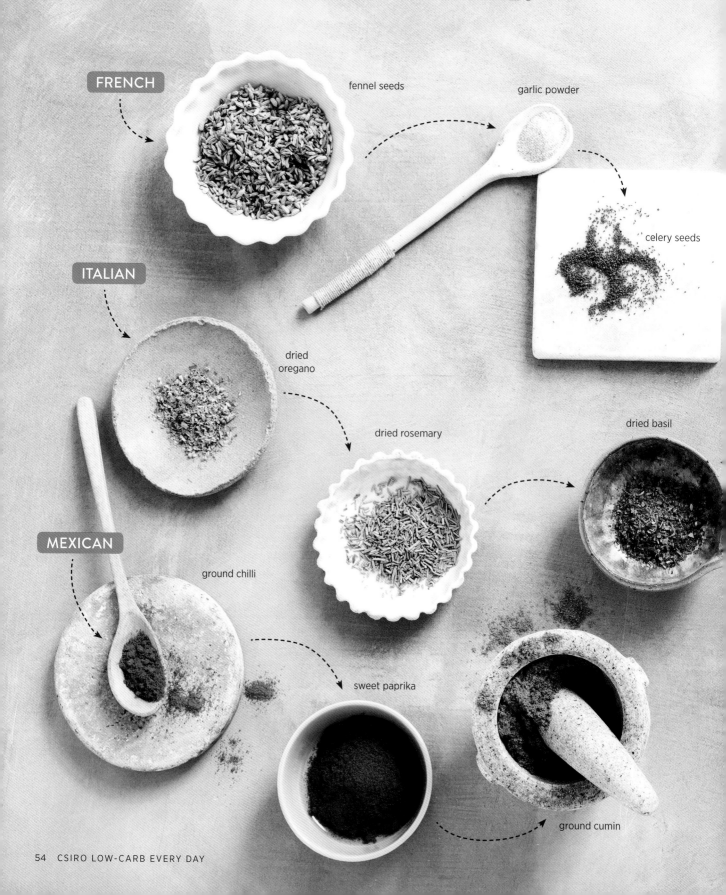

FRENCH

fennel seeds

garlic powder

celery seeds

ITALIAN

dried oregano

dried rosemary

dried basil

MEXICAN

ground chilli

sweet paprika

ground cumin

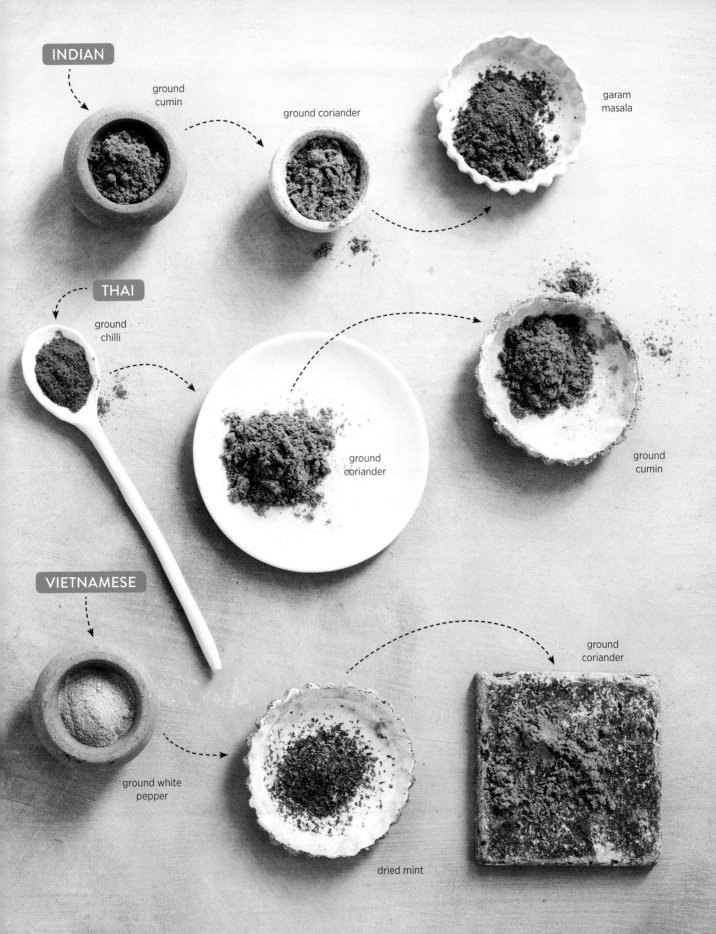

INDIAN

ground cumin

ground coriander

garam masala

THAI

ground chilli

ground coriander

ground cumin

VIETNAMESE

ground white pepper

dried mint

ground coriander

FLAVOUR BOOSTERS: DRESSINGS

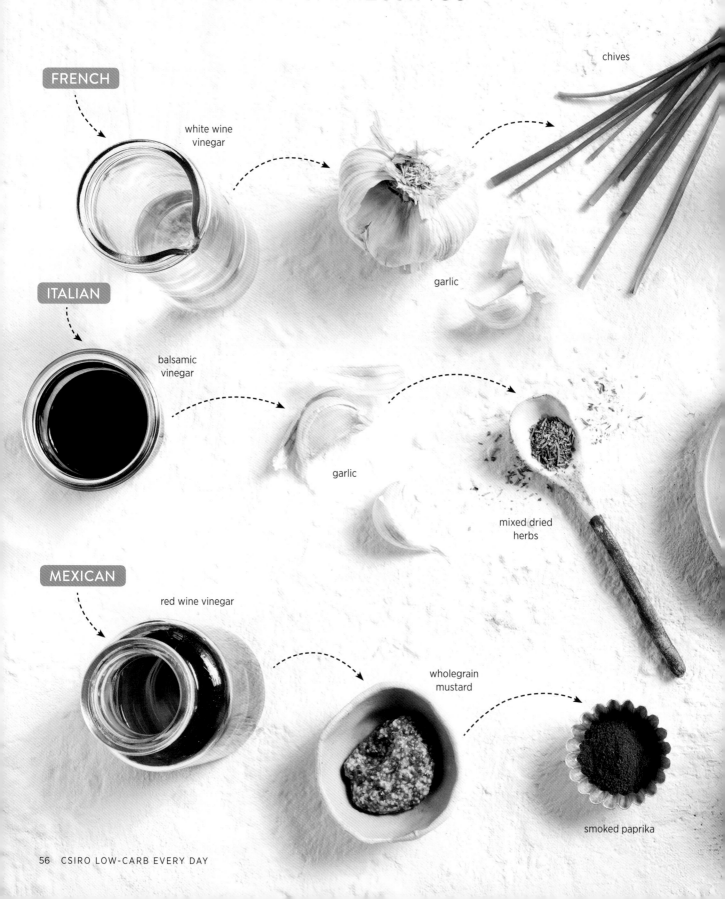

chives

FRENCH

white wine
vinegar

garlic

ITALIAN

balsamic
vinegar

garlic

mixed dried
herbs

MEXICAN

red wine vinegar

wholegrain
mustard

smoked paprika

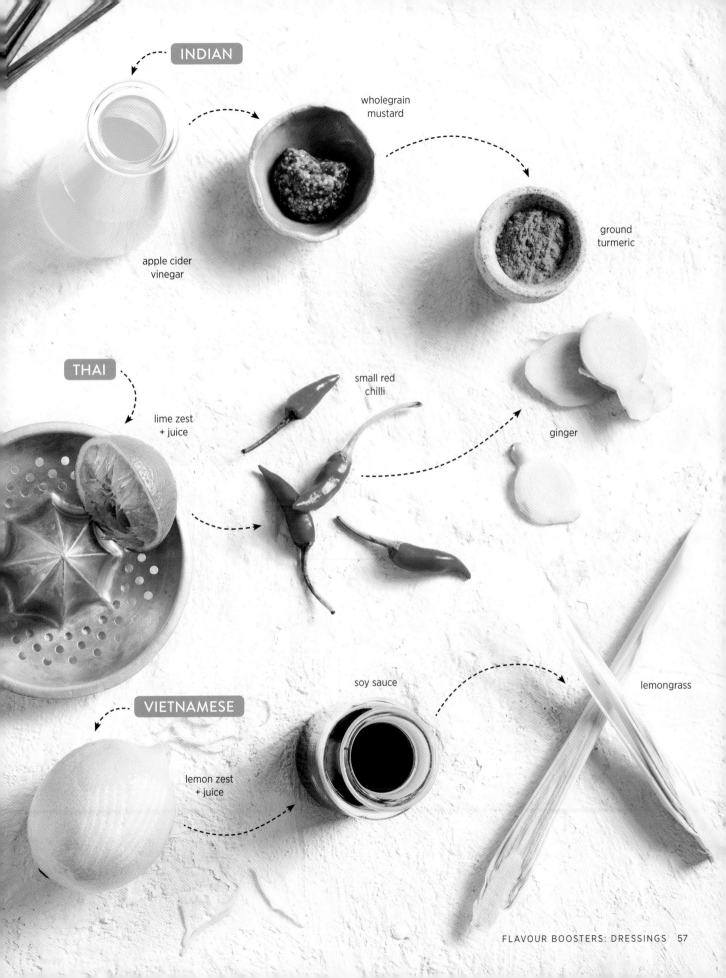

INDIAN

apple cider
vinegar

wholegrain
mustard

ground
turmeric

THAI

lime zest
+ juice

small red
chilli

ginger

soy sauce

lemongrass

VIETNAMESE

lemon zest
+ juice

PART 2

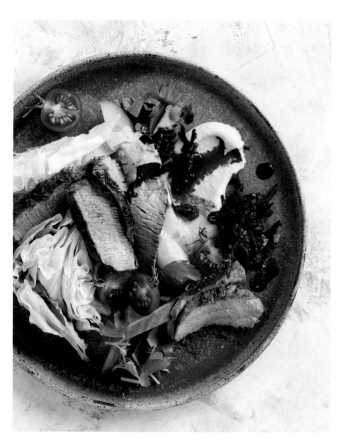

This eating plan offers a way to reduce your intake of carbs while maintaining complete nutrition.

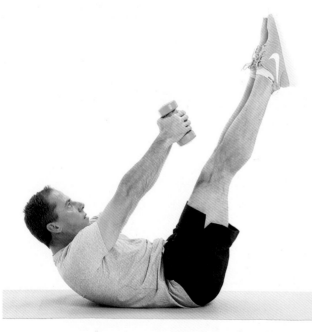

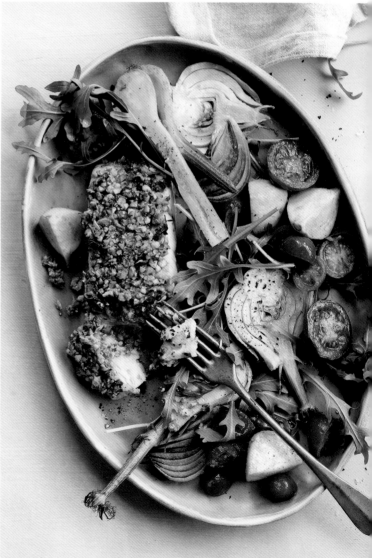

The CSIRO Low-carb Recipes

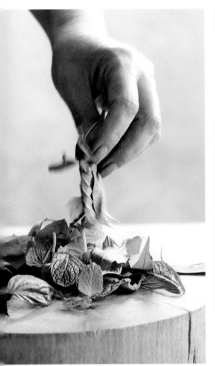
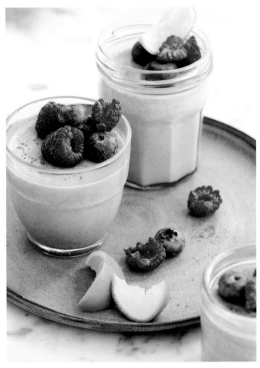
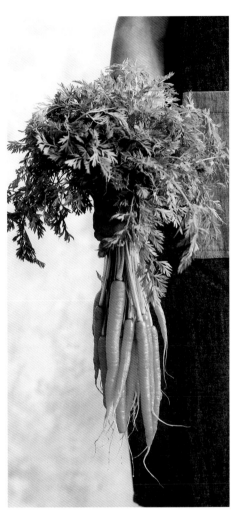
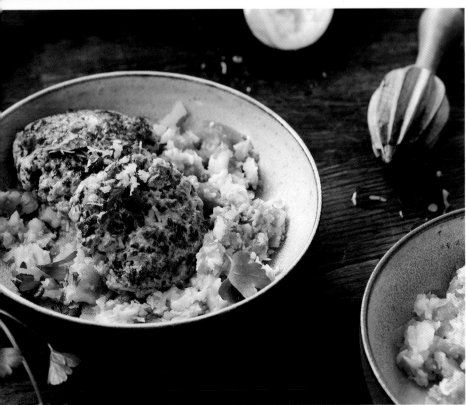

All the recipes have been developed to align with the key principles of the program.

PORTABLE LUNCHES

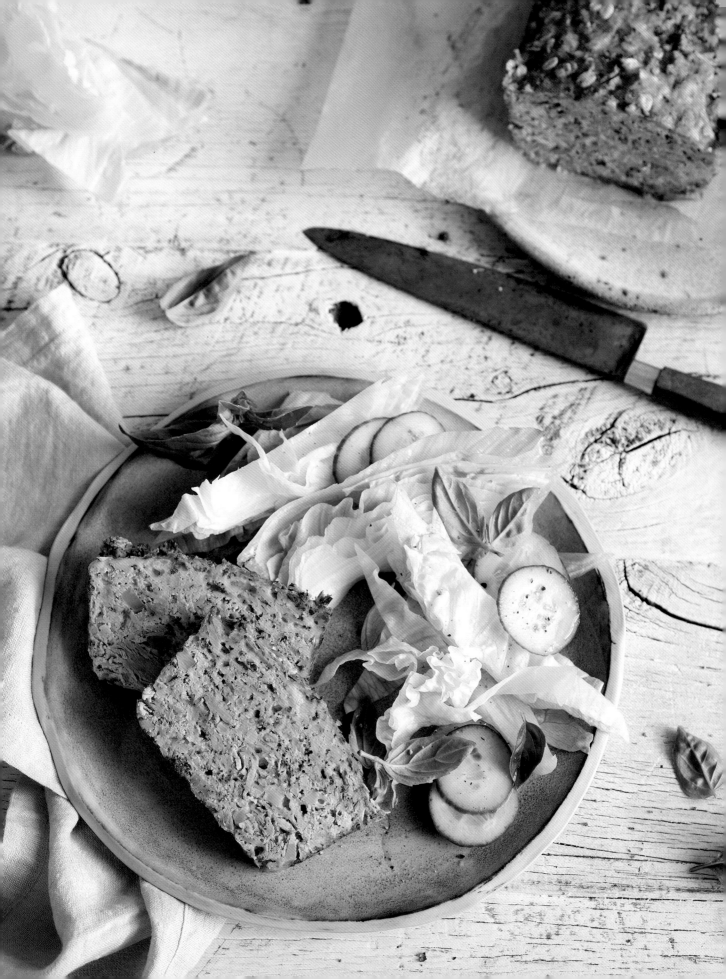

Lean meat, fish, poultry, eggs, tofu: **1**
Breads, cereals, legumes, starchy
    vegetables: **0.5**
Dairy and dairy alternatives: **1**
Low–moderate carb vegetables: **2.5**
Healthy fats: **2**

---

150 g iceberg lettuce, cut into
    thin wedges
150 g Lebanese cucumber, very
    thinly sliced into rounds
1 cup small basil leaves
2 tablespoons white wine vinegar

TUNA LOAF
80 g ground almonds
60 g raw (natural) oats
1 x 425 g tin tuna in springwater,
    drained and flaked
4 eggs, lightly beaten
80 g cheddar, finely grated
150 g broccoli, finely chopped
150 g zucchini, coarsely grated and
    squeezed dry (see note)
2 teaspoons dried mixed herbs

Tuna, cheese and vegetable slice

🍴 **Serves 4**   🕐 **Preparation: 25–30 minutes, plus cooling time**
♨ **Cooking: 45 minutes**   ⓢ **Difficulty: Easy**

Preheat the oven to 200°C (180°C fan-forced). Line the base and sides of an 18 cm x 8 cm loaf tin with baking paper.

To make the tuna loaf, combine all the ingredients in a large bowl and season to taste with freshly ground black pepper. Transfer the mixture to the prepared tin and bake for 45 minutes or until golden and cooked through. Cool in the tin for 10 minutes before slicing.

Place the lettuce, cucumber, basil and vinegar in a bowl. Season to taste with freshly ground black pepper and gently toss together.

Divide the salad and tuna loaf among serving plates and serve.

> **WEEKS 7–12 CARB EXTRAS**
>
> For an extra 6 g carbs per serve, serve with 2 (½ per person) wholemeal mountain bread wraps.

Note: To squeeze the grated zucchini dry, simply place it in a clean tea towel and wring out until all the excess liquid has been released.

 Make it portable: Cool the loaf completely in the tin and wrap tightly before transporting, or cool and slice then transfer to airtight container/s. Place the salad mixture in a separate airtight container. Keep chilled.

UNITS PER SERVE

Lean meat, fish, poultry, eggs, tofu: **1**
Breads, cereals, legumes, starchy
   vegetables: **0.5**
Dairy and dairy alternatives: **1**
Low-moderate carb vegetables: **3**
Healthy fats: **2**

---

400 g lean chicken
   tenderloins, chopped
2 tablespoons chopped tarragon
1 tablespoon thyme leaves
finely grated zest of 1 lemon
2 tablespoons rice bran oil

SUPERGREEN LENTIL SALAD

300 g zucchini, sliced into rounds
150 g broccolini, trimmed
150 g torn kale leaves
juice of 1 lemon
320 g drained and rinsed tinned lentils
½ cup small flat-leaf parsley leaves
100 g cherry bocconcini, torn

Herb chicken patties with supergreen lentil salad

🍴 **Serves 4**　🕐 **Preparation: 30–35 minutes**
🍲 **Cooking: 20 minutes**　👨‍🍳 **Difficulty: Easy**

Place the chicken, tarragon, thyme and lemon zest in a food processor and process until smooth and sticky. Season to taste with freshly ground black pepper. With slightly damp hands, divide the mixture into eight even portions and shape into flat patties. Place on a baking tray lined with baking paper and chill until required.

To make the supergreen lentil salad, preheat a chargrill pan over high heat. Chargrill the zucchini and broccolini, turning occasionally, for 5 minutes or until tender and golden. Transfer to a bowl. Chargrill the kale, turning occasionally, for 1 minute or until crisp and golden. Add to the bowl with the other vegetables. Add the remaining ingredients and season to taste with freshly ground black pepper, then toss well to combine. Set aside until ready to serve.

Heat the rice bran oil in a large frying pan over medium–high heat. Cook the patties, turning occasionally, for 10 minutes or until cooked and golden.

Serve the patties with the supergreen lentil salad.

WEEKS 7–12 CARB EXTRAS

For an extra 8 g carbs per serve, serve with 8 (2 per person) multigrain Ryvita crispbreads.

Make it portable: Cool the patties completely and wrap tightly before transporting or transfer to airtight container/s. Place the salad in a separate airtight container. Keep chilled.

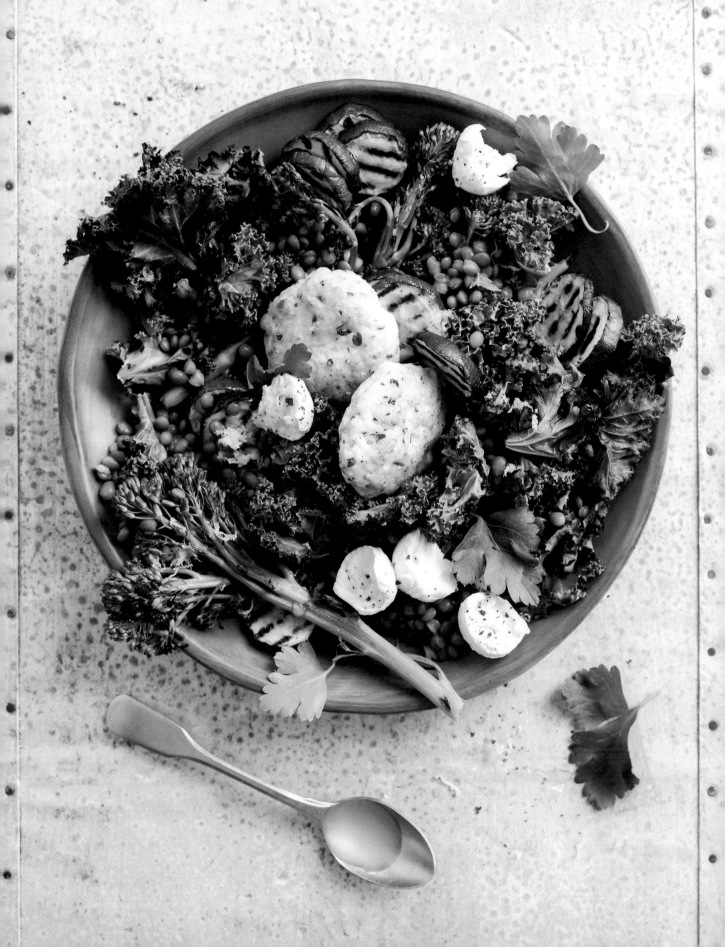

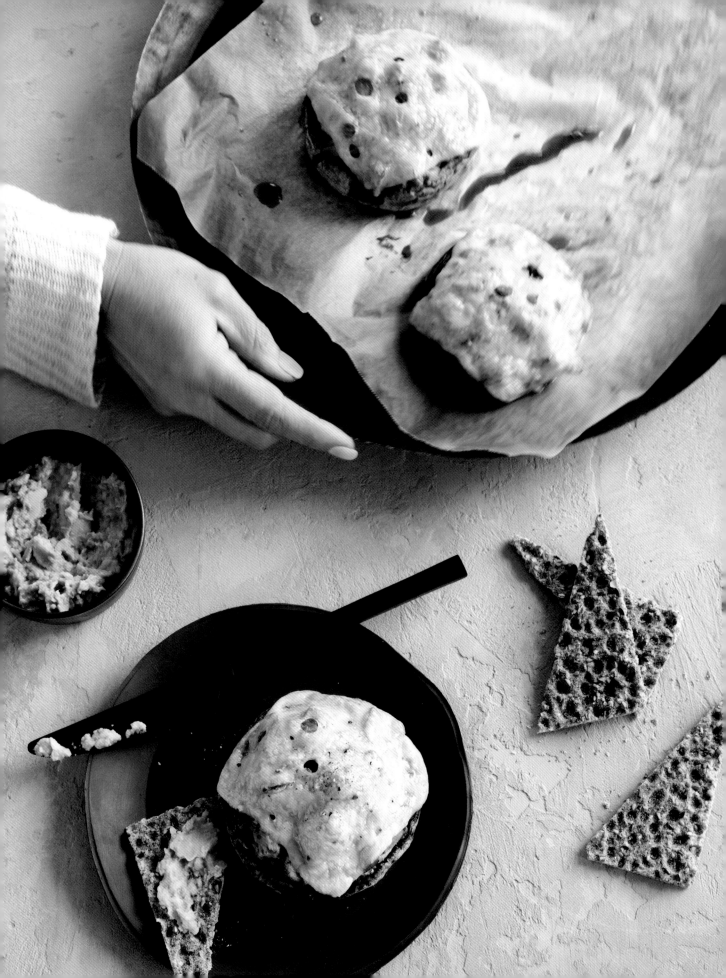

Tuna mushroom melts with avocado crispbreads

UNITS PER SERVE
Lean meat, fish, poultry, eggs, tofu: **1**
Breads, cereals, legumes, starchy
    vegetables: **0.5**
Dairy and dairy alternatives: **1**
Low–moderate carb vegetables: **2.5**
Healthy fats: **2**

🍴 **Serves 4**   🕐 **Preparation: 15–20 minutes**
〰 **Cooking: 10 minutes**   ⏲ **Difficulty: Easy**

1 x 425 g tin tuna in springwater,
    drained, and crushed with a fork
1 clove garlic, crushed
2 teaspoons lemon pepper seasoning
¼ cup chopped flat-leaf parsley
4 field mushrooms (600 g), stems
    removed and finely chopped,
    caps left whole
80 g Swiss cheese, thinly sliced
160 g avocado, mashed
1 tablespoon lemon juice
2 multigrain Ryvita crispbreads,
    halved diagonally

Preheat the oven grill to high.

Combine the tuna, garlic, lemon pepper seasoning, parsley and chopped mushroom stems in a bowl. Season to taste with freshly ground black pepper. Spoon the mixture evenly into the mushroom caps and top with the cheese. Transfer to a baking tray. Cook under the grill for 5–7 minutes or until heated through and the cheese is melted and golden.

Meanwhile, combine the avocado and lemon juice in a bowl. Spread the mixture evenly over the crispbreads and season to taste with freshly ground black pepper.

Serve the mushroom melts with the avocado crispbreads.

WEEKS 7–12 CARB EXTRAS

For an extra 8 g carbs per serve, serve with an extra 8 (2 per person) multigrain Ryvita crispbreads.

Make it portable: Cool the mushrooms completely and transfer to an airtight container for transportation. Place the avocado mixture in a separate airtight container and wrap the crispbreads tightly. Keep them chilled.

15 G
CARB
PER
SERVE

UNITS PER SERVE

Lean meat, fish, poultry, eggs, tofu: **1**
Breads, cereals, legumes, starchy
 vegetables: **0.5**
Dairy and dairy alternatives: **1**
Low–moderate carb vegetables: **4**
Healthy fats: **4**

---

70 g crustless mixed grain bread,
 lightly toasted, chopped
400 g salmon fillet, skin and bones
 removed, flesh chopped
250 g asparagus, trimmed, cut into
 4 cm lengths
1 tablespoon olive oil
1 tablespoon Moroccan spice mix
50 g mixed salad leaves
50 g drained artichoke hearts in brine,
 quartered lengthways
250 g cherry tomatoes,
 sliced into rounds

LOADED HUMMUS

1 tablespoon extra virgin olive oil
160 g hummus
2 tablespoons white wine vinegar
1 tablespoon drained capers in brine,
 rinsed and chopped
2 teaspoons sumac (see note)
2 tablespoons finely chopped basil

Moroccan salmon and crouton salad with loaded hummus

🍴 **Serves 4**   🕐 **Preparation: 20–25 minutes**
🍳 **Cooking: 10 minutes**   ⚙ **Difficulty: Easy**

Preheat the oven to 220°C (200°C fan-forced) and line a large baking tray with baking paper.

To make the loaded hummus, mix together all the ingredients in a bowl and season to taste with freshly ground black pepper. Chill until required.

Combine the bread, salmon, asparagus, olive oil and spice mix in a bowl and season to taste with freshly ground black pepper. Spread out over the prepared tray and bake for 10 minutes or until just cooked and golden.

Meanwhile, combine the salad leaves, artichoke and tomato in a large heatproof bowl. Season to taste with freshly ground black pepper.

Add the hot salmon mixture and any cooking juices to the salad and toss well to combine. Divide among serving plates and serve with the loaded hummus.

WEEKS 7–12 CARB EXTRAS

For an extra 8 g carbs per serve, add an extra 2 slices (½ slice per person) toasted and chopped mixed grain bread, or 1 slice Herman Brot bread per person, to the salmon mixture before baking. (Herman Brot bread provides only 2.5 g carbs per serve, compared to 15 g carbs in a slice of regular bread.)

Note: You can replace the sumac with sweet paprika if preferred.

 Make it portable: Cool the salmon mixture completely before adding to the salad, then transfer to airtight container/s for transportation. Place the loaded hummus in a separate airtight container. Keep chilled.

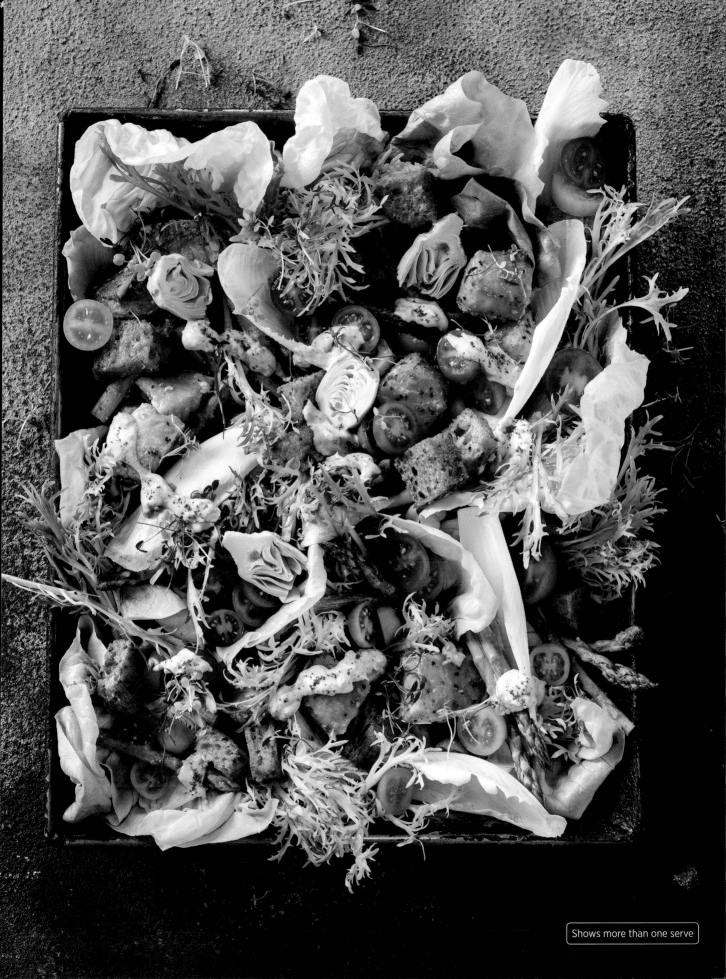

Shows more than one serve

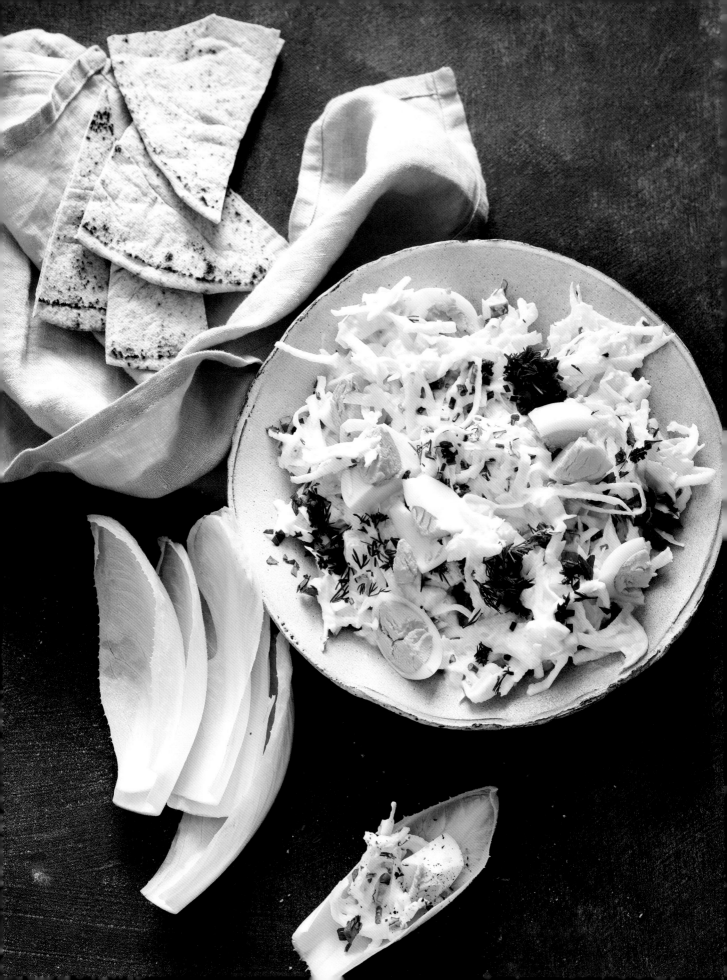

Lean meat, fish, poultry, eggs, tofu: **1**
Breads, cereals, legumes, starchy
vegetables: **0.5**
Dairy and dairy alternatives: **1**
Low–moderate carb vegetables: **2.5**

8 eggs
400 g low-fat natural
  Greek-style yoghurt
2 tablespoons white wine vinegar
150 g Lebanese cucumber,
  finely chopped
300 g peeled celeriac, coarsely grated
2 tablespoons finely chopped
  flat-leaf parsley
2 tablespoons chopped chives
¼ cup dill
150 g green witlof, leaves separated
1 wholemeal pita bread,
  cut into wedges

Creamy celeriac and eggs with witlof

🍴 Serves 4   🕐 Preparation: 20–25 minutes
🍲 Cooking: 10 minutes   👩‍🍳 Difficulty: Easy

Boil the eggs in a large saucepan of boiling water for 8 minutes until hard boiled. Drain and cool, then peel and roughly chop. Transfer to a bowl and set aside.

Place the yoghurt, vinegar, cucumber, celeriac, parsley, chives, dill and ¼ cup (60 ml) water in a bowl and season to taste with freshly ground black pepper. Stir until well combined.

Divide the creamy celeriac among serving plates and top with the egg. Serve with the witlof and pita for scooping.

WEEKS 7–12 CARB EXTRAS

For an extra 7 g carbs per serve, serve with an extra 1 (¼ per person) wholemeal pita bread, or 1 slice Herman Brot bread per person. (Herman Brot bread provides only 2.5 g carbs per serve, compared to 15 g carbs in a slice of regular bread.)

Note: You can replace the celeriac with the same amount of cabbage, and use cos lettuce instead of witlof, if preferred.

Make it portable: Transfer the egg mixture to an airtight container for transportation. Wrap the witlof and pita bread separately. Keep them chilled.

UNITS PER SERVE

Lean meat, fish, poultry, eggs, tofu: **1**

Breads, cereals, legumes, starchy
  vegetables: **1**

Dairy and dairy alternatives: **1**

Low-moderate carb vegetables: **3**

Healthy fats: **4**

---

400 g lean chicken tenderloins
  (see note)

1 wholemeal pita bread

½ cup (125 ml) tomato passata

100 g mozzarella, finely grated

BROCCOLINI AND ROCKET SALAD

1 tablespoon extra virgin olive oil

¼ cup (60 ml) balsamic vinegar

1 teaspoon dried mixed herbs

250 g zucchini, very thinly sliced
  into rounds

300 g broccolini, trimmed

50 g baby rocket leaves

160 g avocado, sliced

40 g slivered almonds, toasted

Chicken pita pizza with broccolini and rocket salad

🍴 **Serves 4** 🕐 **Preparation: 20–25 minutes**
🍳 **Cooking: 20 minutes** 🍲 **Difficulty: Easy**

Preheat the oven grill to high.

Cook the chicken under the grill, turning once, for 12 minutes or until golden and cooked through. Transfer to a board and rest for 5 minutes, then thinly slice diagonally. Cover to keep warm.

Place the pita bread on a large baking tray. Spread evenly with passata and top with mozzarella. Cook under the grill for 3–5 minutes or until the bread has warmed through and the cheese is melted and golden.

Meanwhile, to make the broccolini and rocket salad, combine the olive oil, vinegar, mixed herbs and zucchini in a large bowl. Season to taste with freshly ground black pepper. Place the broccolini in a heatproof bowl and cover with boiling water. Stand for 20 seconds, then drain and immediately add to the zucchini mixture and toss to combine. Add the rocket, avocado and almonds and gently toss again.

Top the pizza with the chicken and serve with the broccolini and rocket salad.

Note: If preferred, you can poach the chicken tenderloins in boiling water for 5 minutes or until cooked. Remove and cool, then shred the meat before adding it to the pizza.

 Make it portable: Cool the pizza and the salad mixture completely before transferring to individual airtight container/s for transportation. Keep chilled.

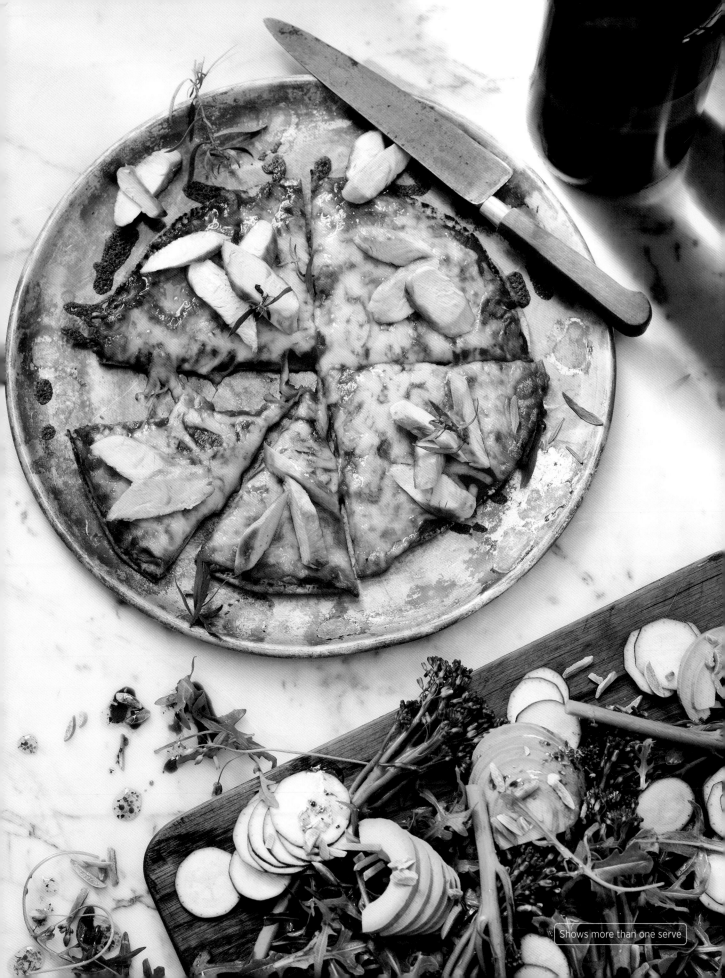

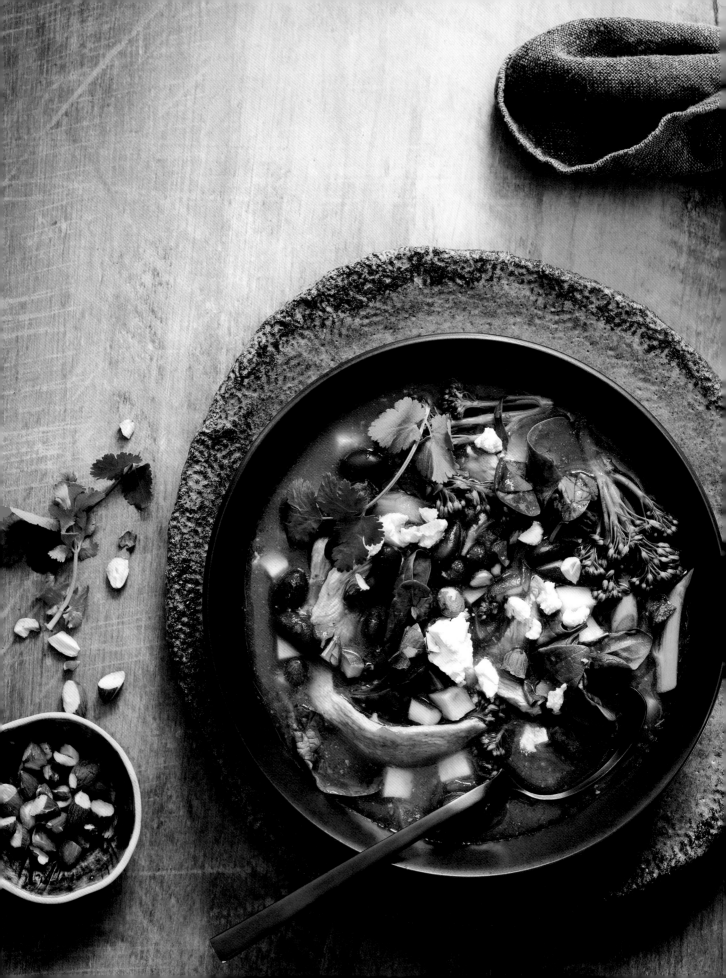

14 G CARB PER SERVE

UNITS PER SERVE

Lean meat, fish, poultry, eggs, tofu: **1**
Breads, cereals, legumes, starchy
   vegetables: **0.5**
Dairy and dairy alternatives: **1**
Low–moderate carb vegetables: **3**
Healthy fats: **2**

400 g lean chicken breast fillets,
   thinly sliced
1 x 300 g jar mild salsa
2 teaspoons Mexican spice mix
160 g drained and rinsed tinned
   red kidney beans
300 g zucchini, finely chopped
1 litre salt-reduced vegetable stock
250 g broccolini, trimmed and cut
   into 3 cm lengths
50 g baby spinach leaves
80 g feta, coarsely crumbled
80 g whole natural almonds,
   toasted and chopped
⅓ cup coriander leaves

Mexican chicken and bean soup

🍴 **Serves 4**   🕐 **Preparation: 15–20 minutes**
♨ **Cooking: 15 minutes**   👨‍🍳 **Difficulty: Easy**

Combine the chicken, salsa, spice mix, kidney beans, zucchini and stock in a large saucepan over medium–high heat. Cook, covered and stirring occasionally, for 15 minutes.

Remove the pan from the heat and stir through the broccolini and spinach until the spinach wilts. Season to taste with freshly ground black pepper.

Divide the soup among serving bowls. Top with the feta, almonds and coriander and serve.

WEEKS 7–12 CARB EXTRAS

For an extra 7 g carbs per serve, add 200 g (50 g per person) peeled and chopped sweet potato to the bean mixture with the other vegetables.

 Make it portable: Cool the soup completely in the pan, then transfer to airtight container/s. Place the feta mixture in an airtight container for transportation. Keep chilled.

Lean meat, fish, poultry, eggs, tofu: **1**
Low–moderate carb vegetables: **3.5**
Healthy fats: **4**

Ginger cashew chicken with edamame zucchini noodles

11 G CARB PER SERVE

🍴 **Serves 4**   🕐 **Preparation: 20–25 minutes**
🍲 **Cooking: 5 minutes**   🎩 **Difficulty: Easy**

2 tablespoons rice bran oil
400 g lean chicken breast
  fillets, chopped
4 cm piece ginger, finely grated
80 g raw unsalted cashews, toasted
  and chopped

EDAMAME ZUCCHINI NOODLES

150 g frozen shelled edamame, thawed
  (see note)
600 g zucchini, spiralised into long
  thin noodles
¼ cup (60 ml) salt-reduced soy sauce
2 tablespoons chopped chives
1 cup small basil leaves

To make the edamame zucchini noodles, combine all the ingredients in a large bowl. Set aside until required.

Heat the rice bran oil in a large wok over high heat. Add the chicken and ginger and stir-fry for 5 minutes or until cooked, crispy and deep golden. Transfer to the zucchini mixture in the bowl and season to taste with freshly ground black pepper. Add the cashews and toss well to combine. Serve.

WEEKS 7–12 CARB EXTRAS

For an extra 6 g carbs per serve, serve with 2 (½ per person) toasted wholemeal mountain bread wraps.

Note: You can buy frozen shelled edamame from Asian supermarkets or buy them in their pods and shell them once the pods have thawed. You will need approximately 250 g edamame pods to produce 150 g shelled edamame.

Replace the basil with Thai basil, if preferred.

Make it portable: Cool the chicken mixture completely and transfer to airtight container/s for transportation. Keep chilled.

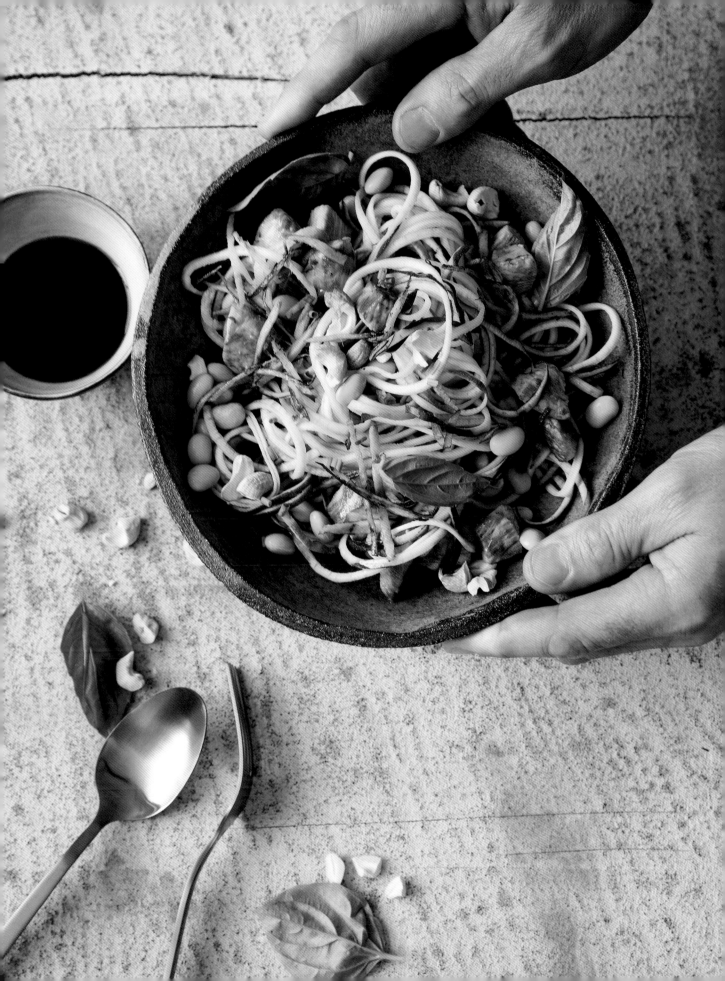

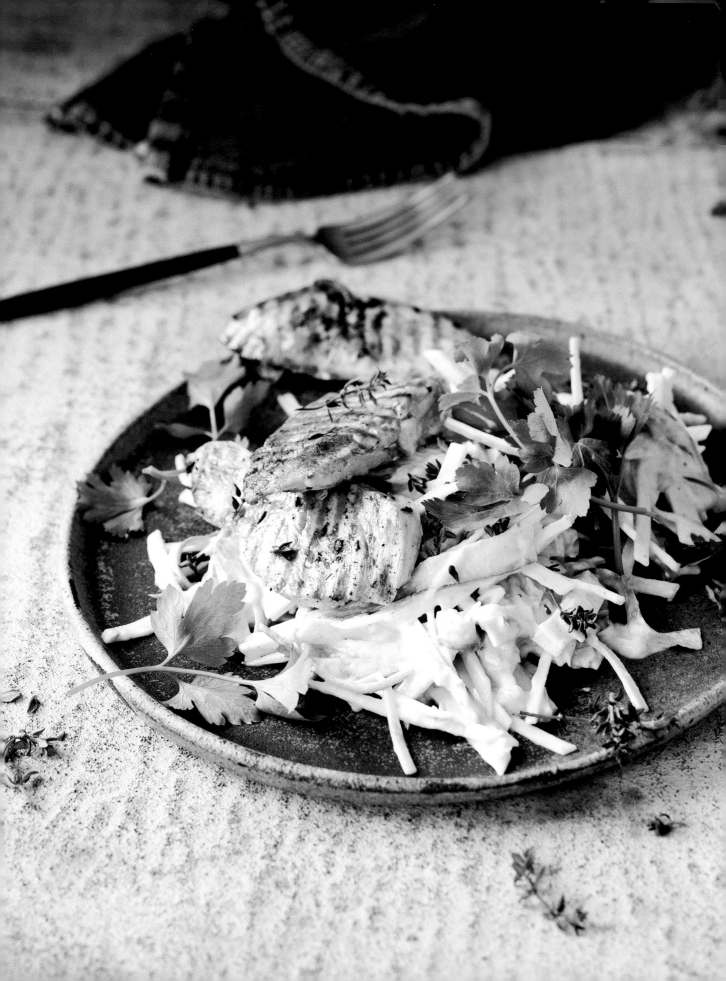

UNITS PER SERVE

Lean meat, fish, poultry, eggs, tofu: **1**
Breads, cereals, legumes, starchy
  vegetables: **0.5**
Dairy and dairy alternatives: **0.5**
Low–moderate carb vegetables: **3**
Healthy fats: **4**

---

400 g lean chicken breast fillets,
  thinly sliced horizontally
1 cup flat-leaf parsley leaves,
  roughly chopped
2 tablespoons thyme leaves

CREAMY CELERIAC SLAW

160 g avocado, chopped
200 g low-fat natural
  Greek-style yoghurt
2 tablespoons tahini
2 tablespoons white wine vinegar
1 teaspoon ground cumin
200 g green apple,
  cut into long thin strips
300 g peeled celeriac,
  cut into long thin strips
300 g Lebanese cucumber,
  cut into long thin strips

Chicken with creamy celeriac slaw

15 G
CARB
PER
SERVE

🍴 **Serves 4**   🕐 **Preparation: 25–30 minutes**
🍳 **Cooking: 5 minutes**   👐 **Difficulty: Easy**

To make the creamy celeriac slaw, mash the avocado in a large bowl until smooth. Add the yoghurt, tahini, vinegar, cumin and ½ cup (125 ml) water and whisk until smooth and well combined. Add the remaining ingredients and season to taste with freshly ground black pepper. Toss gently to combine. Chill until required.

Heat a chargrill pan over high heat.

Season the chicken on both sides with freshly ground black pepper. Cook the chicken on the chargrill for 2 minutes each side or until cooked and golden.

Serve the chargrilled chicken with the creamy celeriac slaw, topped with the parsley and thyme.

> **WEEKS 7–12 CARB EXTRAS**
>
> For an extra 8 g carbs per serve, add 480 g (120 g per person) steamed baby green peas to the slaw.

Note: You could make the slaw with 300 g shredded cabbage and 300 g very finely sliced celery in place of the celeriac and cucumber.

 Make it portable: Cool the chicken completely and wrap tightly before transporting. Place the slaw mixture in an airtight container for transportation. Keep chilled.

UNITS PER SERVE

Lean meat, fish, poultry, eggs, tofu: **1**
Dairy and dairy alternatives: **1**
Low–moderate carb vegetables: **2**
Healthy fats: **5**

Vegetable stuffed egg rolls with macadamia parsley dukkah

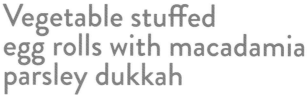

🍽 **Serves 4** 🕐 **Preparation: 25–30 minutes**
🍳 **Cooking: 15 minutes** 👐 **Difficulty: Easy**

8 eggs
1 tablespoon olive oil
80 g avocado, sliced
1 tablespoon apple cider vinegar
150 g Lebanese cucumber, cut into
   long thin strips
225 g asparagus, trimmed and thinly
   sliced lengthways
75 g bean sprouts, trimmed
80 g feta, crumbled
150 g rocket leaves
lemon wedges, to serve

MACADAMIA PARSLEY DUKKAH

1 tablespoon cumin seeds
1 tablespoon coriander seeds
1 tablespoon sesame seeds
80 g macadamias, toasted and
   finely chopped
¼ cup finely chopped flat-leaf
   parsley

Heat a large (22 cm) frying pan over medium–high heat. Whisk two eggs and season to taste with freshly ground black pepper. Heat 1 teaspoon of the olive oil in the hot pan. Add the egg and immediately tilt the pan to make sure it covers the base evenly. Cook, untouched, for 2 minutes. Carefully flip it over and cook for 30 seconds. Slide the omelette out of the pan onto a plate. Cover with a piece of baking paper, then a clean tea towel to keep warm. Repeat with the remaining eggs and oil until you have four omelettes stacked and covered.

To make the macadamia parsley dukkah, dry-fry the cumin, coriander and sesame seeds in a small non-stick frying pan over low heat for 2–3 minutes or until fragrant and lightly golden. Transfer to a small food processor and allow to cool, then process until coarse crumbs form. Add the macadamias and parsley and, using the pulse button, process until just combined. Season to taste with freshly ground black pepper. Set aside until required.

Mash the avocado and vinegar until smooth and well combined. Season to taste with freshly ground black pepper.

Using the baking paper, separate the omelettes and place on your work bench. Top the omelettes evenly with the avocado mixture, cucumber, asparagus, sprouts, feta and rocket. Fold in the sides of each omelette, then roll up firmly to encase the filling. Place, seam-side down, on serving plates and cut in half crossways.

Serve the egg rolls with the macadamia parsley dukkah for dipping and lemon wedges.

WEEKS 7–12 CARB EXTRAS

For an extra 8 g carbs per serve, serve with 8 (2 per person) rye Ryvita crispbreads.

Make it portable: Wrap the omelettes individually before transferring to airtight container/s. Place the dukkah and lemon wedges in separate airtight containers for transportation. Keep chilled.

UNITS PER SERVE

Lean meat, fish, poultry, eggs, tofu: **1**

Breads, cereals, legumes, starchy
vegetables: **0.5**

Dairy and dairy alternatives: **1**

Low–moderate carb vegetables: **2.5**

Healthy fats: **1**

---

8 eggs

220 g cottage cheese

150 g asparagus, trimmed, cut into
4 cm lengths

300 g broccoli florets, chopped

finely grated zest and juice of 1 lemon

⅓ cup dill

1 teaspoon garlic powder

1 teaspoon dried thyme

70 g mixed grain bread, processed
to coarse crumbs

40 g macadamias, finely chopped

rice bran oil spray

50 g mixed salad leaves

100 g cherry tomatoes, sliced
into rounds

2 tablespoons red wine vinegar

Cheesy asparagus and broccoli frittata

🍴 **Serves 4**   🕐 **Preparation: 20–25 minutes**
🍲 **Cooking: 40 minutes**   🍳 **Difficulty: Easy**

Preheat the oven to 200°C (180°C fan-forced). Line the base and side of a 20 cm springform tin with baking paper.

Whisk the eggs and cheese in a large bowl until well combined. Add the asparagus, broccoli, lemon zest and juice, dill, garlic powder and thyme. Season to taste with freshly ground black pepper and stir until well combined. Pour the mixture into the prepared tin and sprinkle the breadcrumbs and chopped macadamia over the top. Spray lightly with rice bran oil.

Bake for 40 minutes or until golden and set in the centre. Rest in the tin for 5 minutes, then carefully remove and cut into wedges.

Combine the salad leaves, tomato and vinegar in a bowl. Divide among serving plates, add the frittata wedges and serve.

> **WEEKS 7–12 CARB EXTRAS**
>
> For an extra 9 g carbs per serve, add 160 g (40 g per person) cooked puy lentils to the salad mixture before serving.

 Make it portable: Cool the frittata completely in the tin and wrap tightly before transporting, or cool and slice then transfer to individual airtight container/s. Place the salad in an airtight container for transportation. Keep chilled.

Lean meat, fish, poultry, eggs, tofu: **1**
Low–moderate carb vegetables: **2**
Healthy fats: **4**

Tofu and edamame san choy bau

11 G CARB PER SERVE

🍴 **Serves 4**   🕐 **Preparation: 15–20 minutes**
🍲 **Cooking: 10 minutes**   👩‍🍳 **Difficulty: Easy**

2 tablespoons rice bran oil
1 teaspoon sesame oil
400 g firm tofu, finely chopped
150 g frozen shelled edamame, thawed
  (see note)
150 g mixed mushrooms, torn
2 cloves garlic, crushed
1 fresh long red chilli, finely chopped
⅓ cup (80 ml) oyster sauce
2 tablespoons chopped chives
300 g baby cos lettuce,
  leaves separated
80 g blanched almonds, toasted
  and finely chopped

Heat the oils in a large wok over high heat. Add the tofu and stir-fry for 4 minutes or until crispy and golden. Add the edamame, mushrooms, garlic and chilli and stir-fry for 2 minutes.

Add the oyster sauce and ⅓ cup (80 ml) water and stir-fry for 1 minute or until well combined and coated. Remove the wok from the heat and toss the chives through.

Divide the cos leaves among serving plates. Fill with the tofu mixture, sprinkle with the chopped almonds and season to taste with freshly ground black pepper. Serve.

WEEKS 7–12 CARB EXTRAS

For an extra 8 g carbs per serve, toss 200 g (50 g per person) cooked quinoa through the tofu mixture before serving.

Note: You can buy frozen shelled edamame from Asian supermarkets or buy them in their pods and shell them once the pods have thawed. You will need approximately 250 g edamame pods to produce 150 g shelled edamame.

Make it portable: Cool the tofu mixture completely and transfer to airtight container/s. Place the lettuce leaves and chopped almonds in separate airtight containers for transportation. Keep chilled.

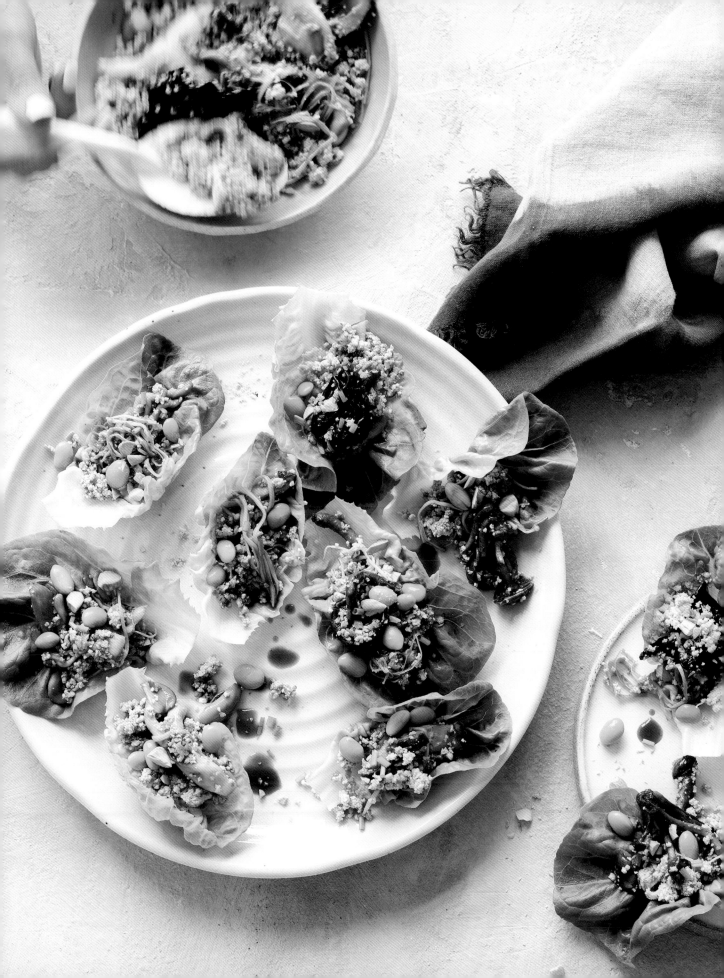

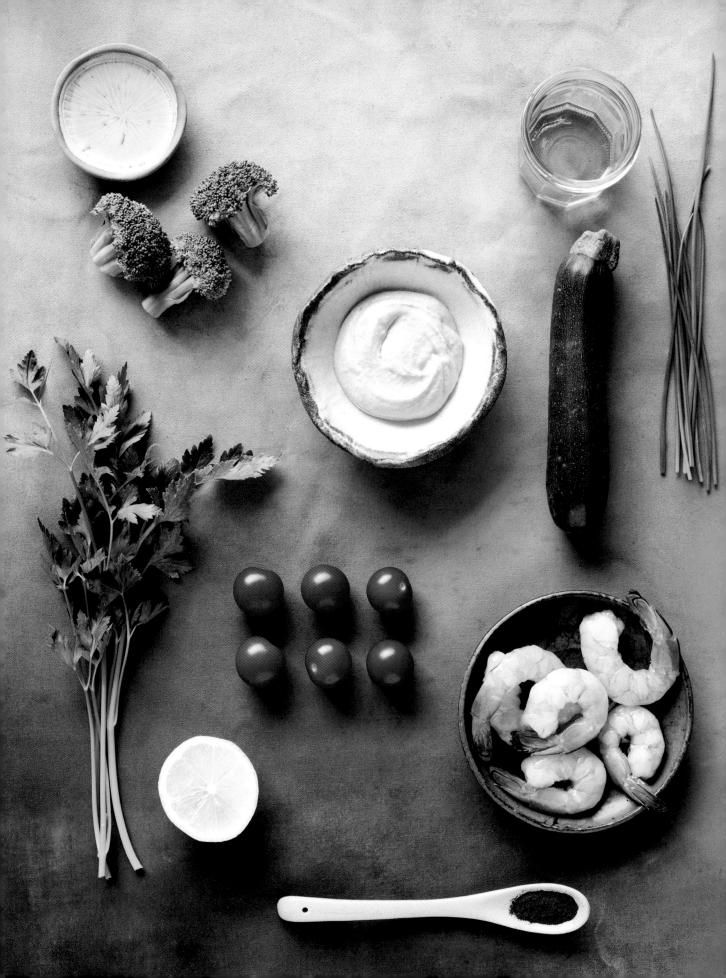

UNITS PER SERVE
Lean meat, fish, poultry, eggs, tofu: **1**
Low–moderate carb vegetables: **2**
Healthy fats: **4**

Prawns with zucchini and broccoli tabouleh

8 G CARB PER SERVE

🍽 Serves 4   🕐 Preparation: 20–25 minutes
🍲 Cooking: 10 minutes   👨‍🍳 Difficulty: Easy

1 tablespoon rice bran oil
400 g peeled, deveined raw king
  prawns, tails left on
1 tablespoon smoked paprika
⅔ cup (160 g) hummus

ZUCCHINI AND BROCCOLI TABOULEH
150 g zucchini
300 g broccoli florets
150 g sweet cherry tomatoes,
  finely chopped
1 tablespoon extra virgin olive oil
finely grated zest and juice of 1 lemon
¼ cup chopped chives
½ cup finely chopped flat-leaf parsley

To make the zucchini and broccoli tabouleh, process the zucchini and broccoli separately in a food processor until finely chopped. Place in a large bowl. Add all the remaining ingredients and season to taste with freshly ground black pepper. Set aside until required.

Heat a chargrill pan over high heat. Combine the rice bran oil, prawns and paprika in a bowl and season to taste with freshly ground black pepper. Chargrill the prawns, turning occasionally, for 6 minutes or until cooked and golden.

Divide the zucchini and broccoli tabouleh among serving plates. Top with the prawns and hummus and serve.

WEEKS 7–12 CARB EXTRAS

For an extra 8 g carbs per serve, serve with 200 g (50 g per person) cooked quinoa.

Make it portable: Cool the prawns completely, then transfer to individual airtight container/s. Place the tabouleh mixture in an airtight container for transportation. Keep chilled.

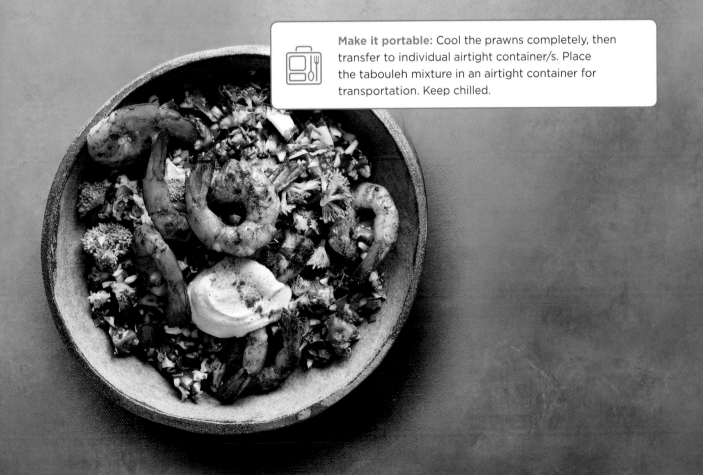

UNITS PER SERVE

Lean meat, fish, poultry, eggs, tofu: **1**
Low–moderate carb vegetables: **2**
Healthy fats: **4**

Vietnamese prawn salad with almond dressing

6 G CARB PER SERVE

🍴 **Serves 4**   🕐 **Preparation: 20–25 minutes**
🍲 **Cooking: 5 minutes**   ⓦ **Difficulty: Easy**

1 tablespoon rice bran oil
2 stalks lemongrass, white part only, very finely chopped
400 g peeled, deveined raw king prawns, tails left on
200 g butter lettuce, torn
75 g bean sprouts
225 g Lebanese cucumbers, very thinly sliced diagonally
100 g asparagus, trimmed, shaved lengthways with a vegetable peeler
1 cup small Vietnamese mint leaves (see note)
1 cup small coriander sprigs

ALMOND DRESSING

finely grated zest and juice of 2 limes
1 fresh long red chilli, finely chopped
¼ cup (60 ml) salt-reduced soy sauce
1 tablespoon extra virgin olive oil
80 g blanched almonds, toasted and finely chopped

To make the almond dressing, mix together all the ingredients in a small bowl and season to taste with freshly ground black pepper. Set aside until required.

Heat the rice bran oil in a large wok over high heat. Add the lemongrass and prawns and stir-fry for 3–4 minutes or until cooked and golden. Transfer to a bowl, cover loosely with foil and rest for 3 minutes.

Meanwhile, combine the lettuce, sprouts, cucumber, asparagus, mint and coriander in a large bowl.

Divide the salad among serving plates and top with the prawns and any juices. Spoon over the almond dressing and serve.

WEEKS 7–12 CARB EXTRAS

For an extra 7 g carbs per serve, serve with 2 (½ per person) toasted wholemeal mountain bread wraps.

Note: You can swap regular mint for Vietnamese mint, if desired.

 Make it portable: Cool the prawns completely, then toss with the salad mixture and transfer to airtight container/s. Place the dressing in a separate airtight container for transportation. Keep chilled.

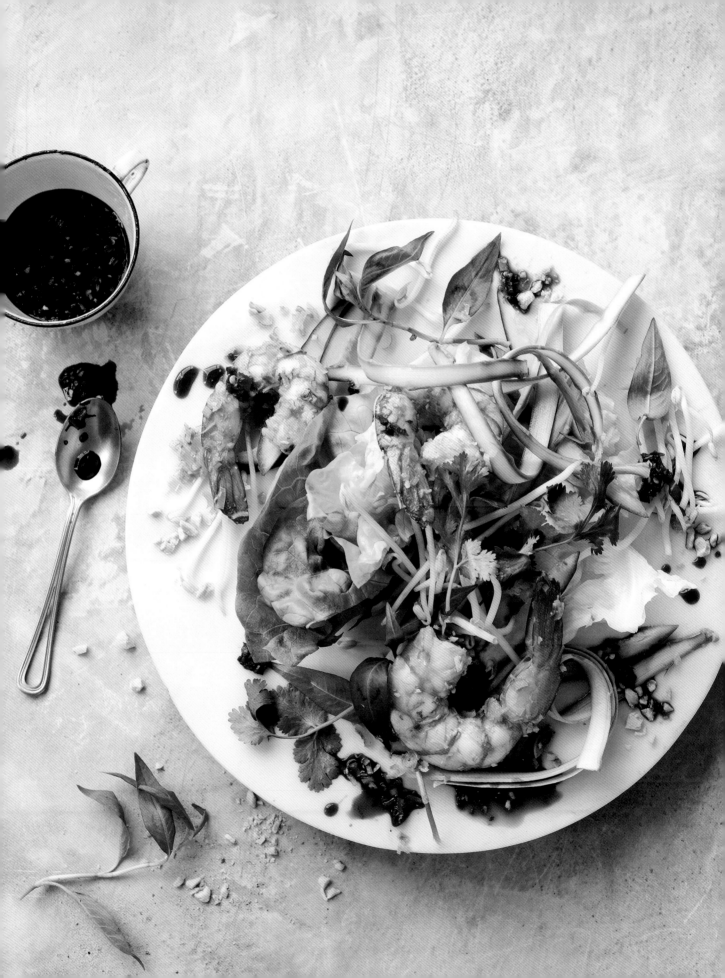

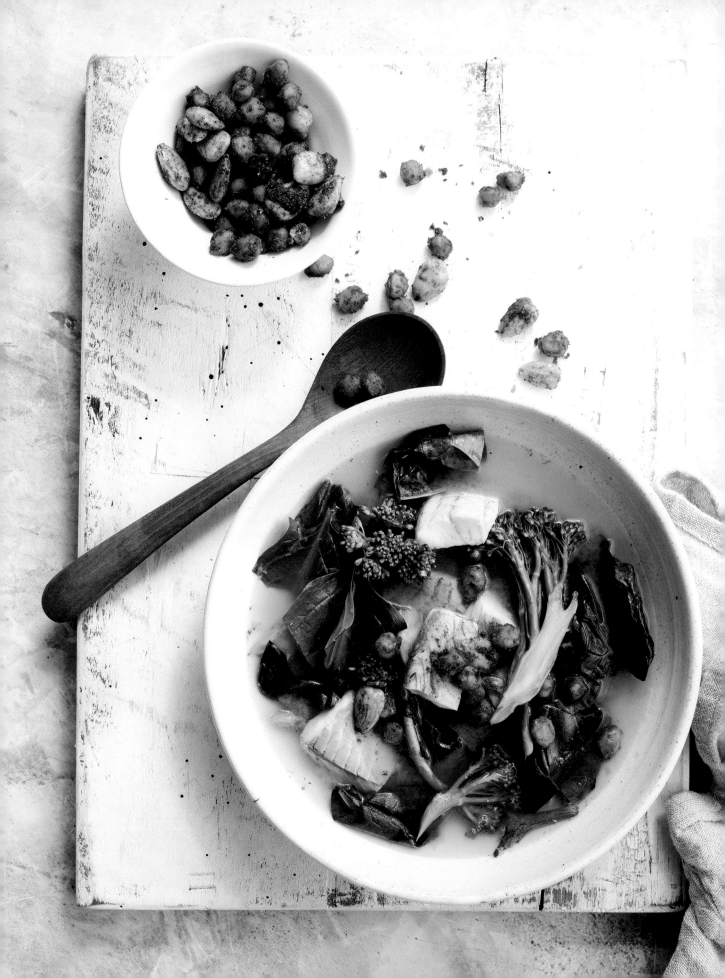

Fish and greens soup with curried chickpeas and almonds

UNITS PER SERVE

Lean meat, fish, poultry, eggs, tofu: **1**
Breads, cereals, legumes, starchy
   vegetables: **0.5**
Low–moderate carb vegetables: **2**
Healthy fats: **4**

🍽 **Serves 4**   🕐 **Preparation: 20–25 minutes**
♨ **Cooking: 25 minutes**   👨‍🍳 **Difficulty: Easy**

400 g flathead fillets, skin and bones
   removed, cut into 5 cm pieces
2 cloves garlic, crushed
2 cm piece ginger, finely grated
1 cinnamon stick, broken in half
1 litre salt-reduced chicken stock
300 g broccolini, trimmed, halved
   lengthways and cut into 5 cm lengths
300 g English spinach leaves,
   thickly sliced
finely grated zest and juice of 1 lemon

CURRIED CHICKPEAS AND ALMONDS

160 g drained and rinsed tinned
   chickpeas, patted dry
1 tablespoon olive oil
1 tablespoon curry powder
120 g blanched almonds

To make the curried chickpeas and almonds, preheat the oven to 220°C (200°C fan-forced) and line a baking tray with baking paper. Combine the chickpeas, olive oil and curry powder in a bowl and season to taste with freshly ground black pepper. Spread the mixture evenly over the prepared tray and roast for 20 minutes. Add the almonds and roast for a further 5 minutes or until the mixture is crisp and golden. Set aside until required.

Meanwhile, place the flathead, garlic, ginger, cinnamon, stock, broccolini and spinach in a large saucepan over medium–high heat. Cook, covered and shaking the pan occasionally, for 15 minutes or until the fish is cooked through and the stock has reduced slightly. Remove the pan from the heat and stir through the lemon zest and juice. Remove and discard the cinnamon.

Divide the soup among serving bowls and serve with the curried chickpeas and almonds.

WEEKS 7–12 CARB EXTRAS

For an extra 8 g carbs per serve, add 200 g (50 g per person) peeled and diced sweet potato to the fish mixture when cooking.

Make it portable: Cool the soup completely in the pan then transfer to airtight container/s. Place the cooled chickpea mixture in an airtight container for transportation. Keep chilled.

UNITS PER SERVE
Lean meat, fish, poultry, eggs, tofu: **1**
Low–moderate carb vegetables: **2.5**
Healthy fats: **4**

Sesame-crusted hoisin tofu steaks

12 G CARB PER SERVE

🍽 Serves 4　🕐 Preparation: 25–30 minutes
♨ Cooking: 10 minutes　🎛 Difficulty: Easy

400 g piece firm tofu, cut into
　four even pieces
2 tablespoons hoisin sauce
1 tablespoon salt-reduced soy sauce
40 g sesame seeds
1 tablespoon rice bran oil
80 g avocado, sliced
½ cup basil sprigs
¼ cup coriander sprigs
lime wedges, to serve

**BROCCOLI RICE AND
BOK CHOY**

300 g baby bok choy, leaves separated
300 g broccoli florets
40 g raw unsalted cashews, toasted
　and chopped

To make the broccoli rice and bok choy, place the bok choy in a large heatproof bowl and cover with boiling water. Stand for 1 minute, then drain and rinse under cold running water. Transfer to a large bowl. Process the broccoli in a food processor until it resembles rice grains. Add to the bok choy. Add the cashews and season to taste with freshly ground black pepper, then toss until well combined.

Coat the tofu pieces in the hoisin and soy sauces, then press firmly into the sesame seeds on all sides. Heat the rice bran oil in a large frying pan over medium heat. Add the tofu and cook, turning occasionally, for 6 minutes or until heated through, crisp and golden. Transfer to a plate and cover to keep warm. Add ½ cup (125 ml) water to the pan and swirl it around for 30 seconds, scraping the base to release the flavourings. Transfer to a heatproof jug.

Meanwhile, gently combine the avocado, basil and coriander in a bowl. Season to taste with freshly ground black pepper.

Divide the broccoli rice among serving plates. Top with the tofu steaks and drizzle with the sauce mixture from the pan. Serve with the avocado and herb salad and lime wedges.

WEEKS 7–12 CARB EXTRAS

For an extra 8 g carbs per serve, serve with 2 slices (½ slice per person) toasted mixed grain bread.

Make it portable: Cool the tofu completely, then transfer to airtight container/s, along with the sauce from the pan. Place the broccoli rice and the avocado salad in separate airtight containers for transportation. Keep chilled.

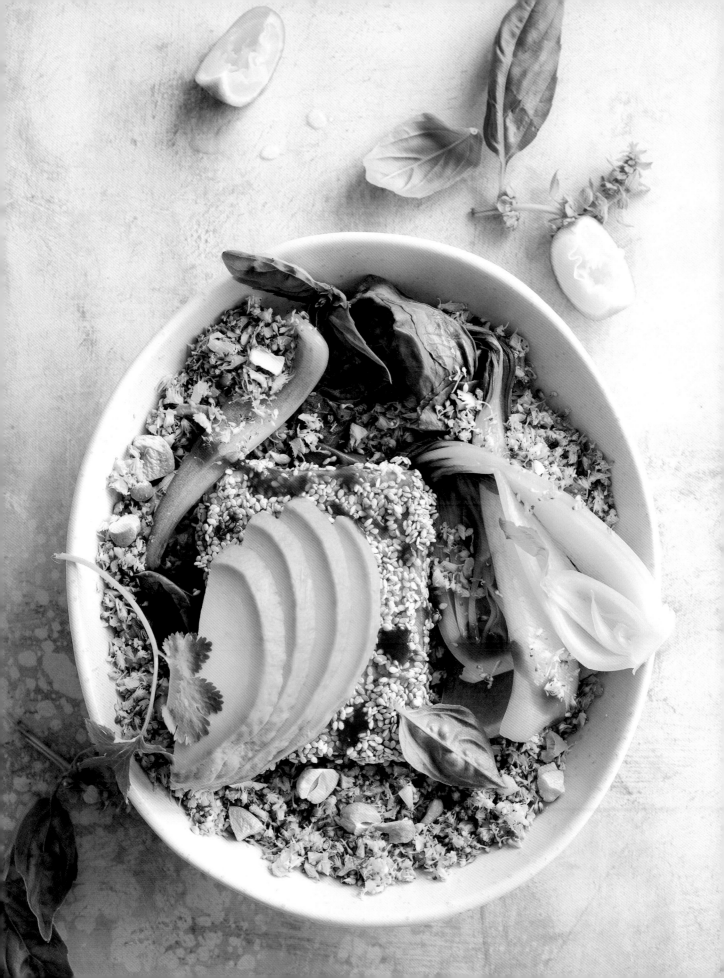

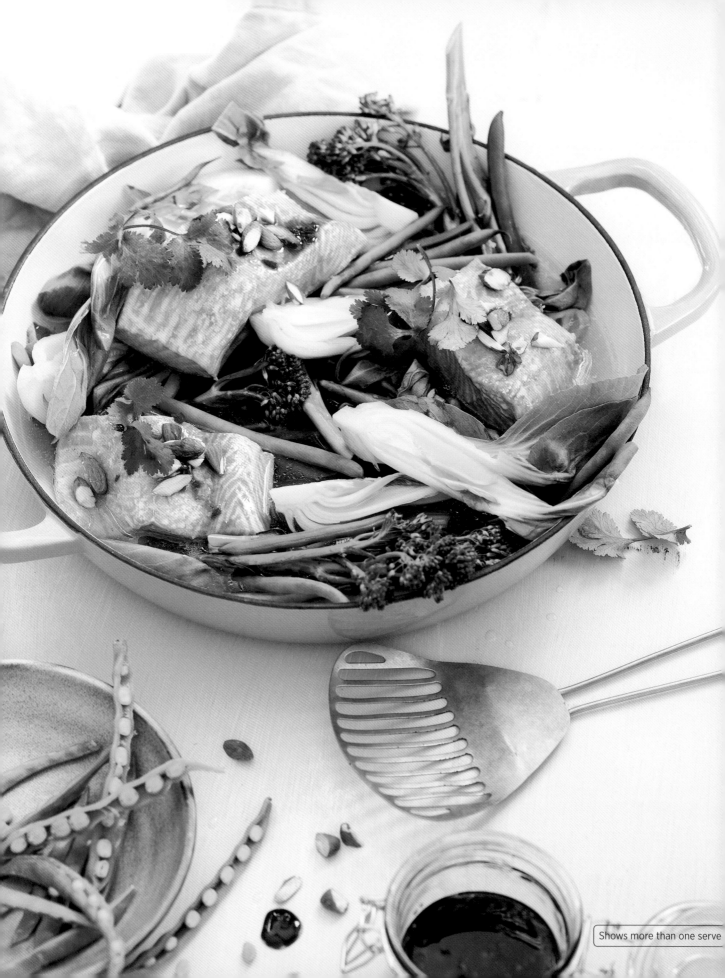

UNITS PER SERVE

Lean meat, fish, poultry, eggs, tofu: **1.5**
Low–moderate carb vegetables: **4**
Healthy fats: **1.5**

One-pan chilli-soy salmon

6 G
CARB
PER
SERVE

🍴 **Serves 4**　🕐 **Preparation: 20–25 minutes**
🍲 **Cooking: 10 minutes**　🍳 **Difficulty: Easy**

⅓ cup (80 ml) salt-reduced soy sauce
1 teaspoon sesame oil
1 small fresh red chilli, finely chopped
1 clove garlic, crushed
3 cups (750 ml) salt-reduced
　chicken stock
150 g green beans, trimmed
300 g broccolini, trimmed and
　halved lengthways
300 g baby bok choy,
　quartered lengthways
4 x 150 g salmon fillets, skin on,
　bones removed
150 g snow peas, halved lengthways
½ cup small coriander sprigs
50 g whole natural almonds, toasted
　and chopped

Combine the soy sauce, sesame oil, chilli and garlic in a small jug. Season to taste with freshly ground black pepper.

Place the stock, beans and broccolini in a large deep frying pan over high heat and bring to the boil. Add the bok choy and rest the salmon fillets on top, then pour the soy sauce mixture over the salmon. Cover and cook, untouched, for 6 minutes for medium or until the salmon is cooked to your liking.

Meanwhile, divide the snow peas among serving bowls.

Spoon the salmon and vegetables over the snow peas. Top with the coriander and almonds and serve.

WEEKS 7–12 CARB EXTRAS

For an extra 12 g carbs per serve, serve with 160 g (40 g per person) cooked brown basmati rice.

Roast Moroccan chicken with lemony herbed feta

UNITS PER SERVE
Lean meat, fish, poultry, eggs, tofu: **1.5**
Dairy and dairy alternatives: **2**
Low–moderate carb vegetables: **3**

⑪ Serves 4   **⏲ Preparation: 15–20 minutes**
⊛ Cooking: 15 minutes   **⑨ Difficulty: Easy**

600 g lean chicken tenderloins,
    halved diagonally
300 g zucchini, halved lengthways,
    sliced diagonally
300 g small cauliflower florets
300 g cherry tomatoes
1 tablespoon Moroccan seasoning
1 cup (250 ml) salt-reduced
    chicken stock

LEMONY HERBED FETA
finely grated zest and juice of 1 lemon
¾ cup flat-leaf parsley leaves
¾ cup coriander leaves
1 small clove garlic, crushed
160 g feta, coarsely crumbled

Preheat the oven to 220°C (200°C fan-forced). Place a heavy-based baking dish in the oven to heat while you prepare your ingredients.

To make the lemony herbed feta, place all the ingredients in a bowl and mix together with a fork. Season to taste with freshly ground black pepper. Set aside until required.

Combine the chicken, zucchini, cauliflower, tomatoes, seasoning and stock in a large bowl and season to taste with freshly ground black pepper. Carefully remove the hot dish from the oven. Add the chicken mixture, then shake the dish to spread the mixture evenly over the base. Roast for 15 minutes or until the chicken and vegetables are cooked and tender.

Remove the dish from the oven. Scatter the lemony herbed feta over the top and serve.

WEEKS 7–12 CARB EXTRAS

For an extra 7–9 g carbs per serve, serve with 200 g (50 g per person) peeled, steamed and mashed sweet potato or cooked quinoa.

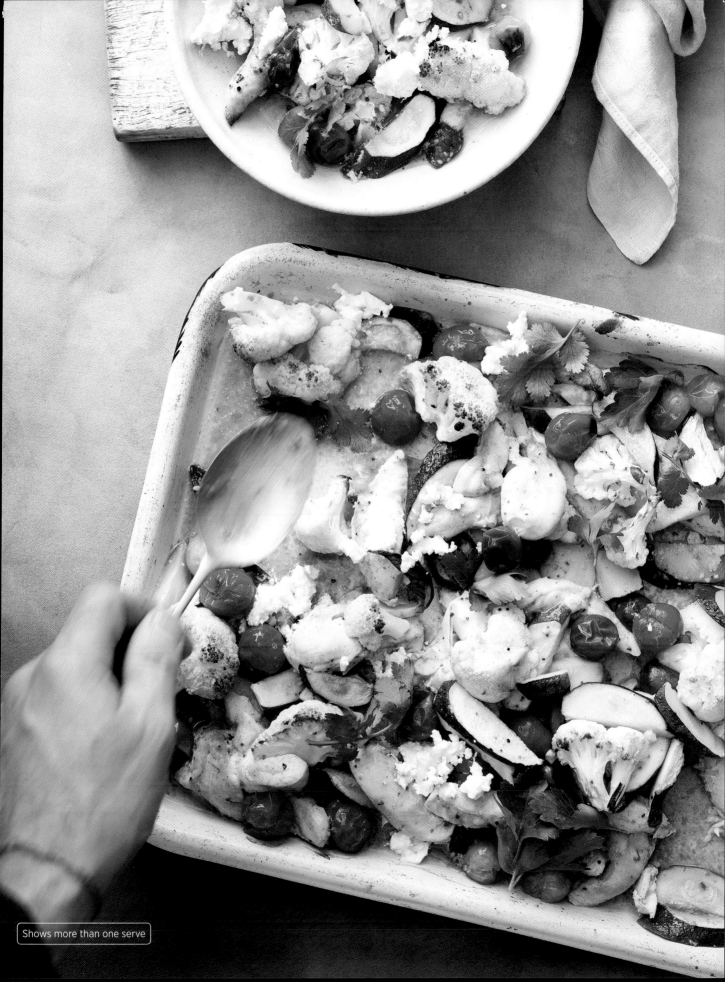

Shows more than one serve

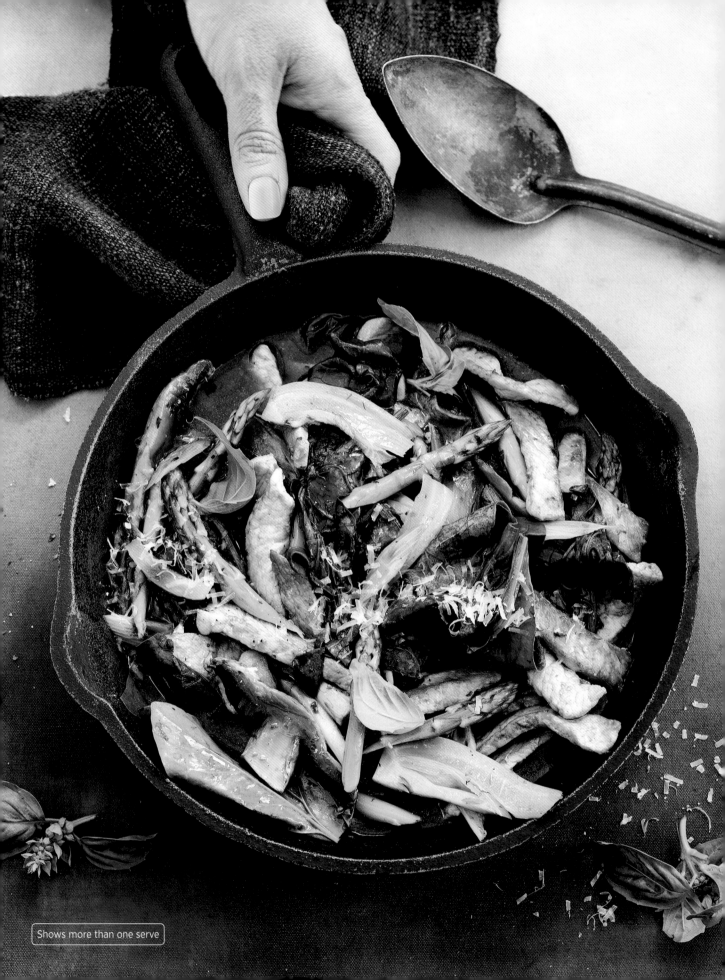

Shows more than one serve

One-pan pork and Italian vegetables

UNITS PER SERVE

Lean meat, fish, poultry, eggs, tofu: **1.5**
Dairy and dairy alternatives: **1**
Low–moderate carb vegetables: **3.5**
Healthy fats: **2**

🍴 **Serves 4**   🕐 **Preparation: 15–20 minutes**
🍲 **Cooking: 10 minutes**   🎩 **Difficulty: Easy**

1 tablespoon extra virgin olive oil
600 g lean pork leg steaks, thinly sliced
300 g cap mushrooms, thickly sliced
2 cloves garlic, crushed
2 teaspoons dried mixed herbs
300 g baby fennel, thinly sliced
2 cups (500 ml) salt-reduced
  vegetable stock
150 g asparagus, trimmed and
  halved crossways
150 g English spinach, trimmed,
  leaves torn in half
1 cup small basil leaves
80 g parmesan, finely grated

Heat the olive oil in a large saucepan over high heat. Add the pork, mushroom, garlic, dried mixed herbs and fennel and cook, stirring occasionally, for 5 minutes. Add the stock and cook, stirring occasionally, for 2 minutes. Add the asparagus and spinach and cook, stirring, for 3 minutes or until the vegetables are tender, the pork is cooked through and the stock has reduced by half.

Remove the pan from the heat. Stir through the basil and season to taste with freshly ground black pepper. Serve topped with the parmesan.

WEEKS 7–12 CARB EXTRAS

For an extra 4 g carbs per serve, add 200 g (50 g per person) drained and rinsed tinned butter beans to the pan in the last 5 minutes of cooking.

Note: You could add 16 pitted Sicilian green olives (4 per person) before serving.

UNITS PER SERVE

Lean meat, fish, poultry, eggs, tofu: **1.5**
Low–moderate carb vegetables: **2.5**
Healthy fats: **4**

Grilled lamb with mint dressing

5 G
CARB
PER
SERVE

1 tablespoon extra virgin olive oil
2 teaspoons sumac
1 clove garlic, crushed
300 g asparagus, trimmed
300 g small vine-ripened tomatoes
600 g French-trimmed lamb cutlets
150 g rocket leaves
150 g Lebanese cucumber, cut
   with a vegetable peeler into
   long thin ribbons
160 g avocado, sliced

MINT DRESSING

1 tablespoon extra virgin olive oil
½ cup (125 ml) apple cider vinegar
⅓ cup finely chopped mint

🍴 **Serves 4**   🕐 **Preparation: 20–25 minutes**
🍳 **Cooking: 15 minutes**   🍲 **Difficulty: Easy**

Preheat the oven grill to high. Place a large baking tray under the grill to preheat.

To make the mint dressing, whisk together all the ingredients in a small jug and season to taste with freshly ground black pepper. Set aside until required.

Combine the olive oil, sumac, garlic, asparagus, tomatoes and lamb in a large bowl and season to taste with freshly ground black pepper. Carefully spread the mixture over the preheated tray. Grill, untouched, for 10–12 minutes or until cooked and golden.

Divide the lamb and vegetable mixture among serving plates and add the rocket, cucumber and avocado. Spoon over the mint dressing and serve.

WEEKS 7–12 CARB EXTRAS

For an extra 7 g carbs per serve, serve with 2 (½ per person) wholemeal pita breads.

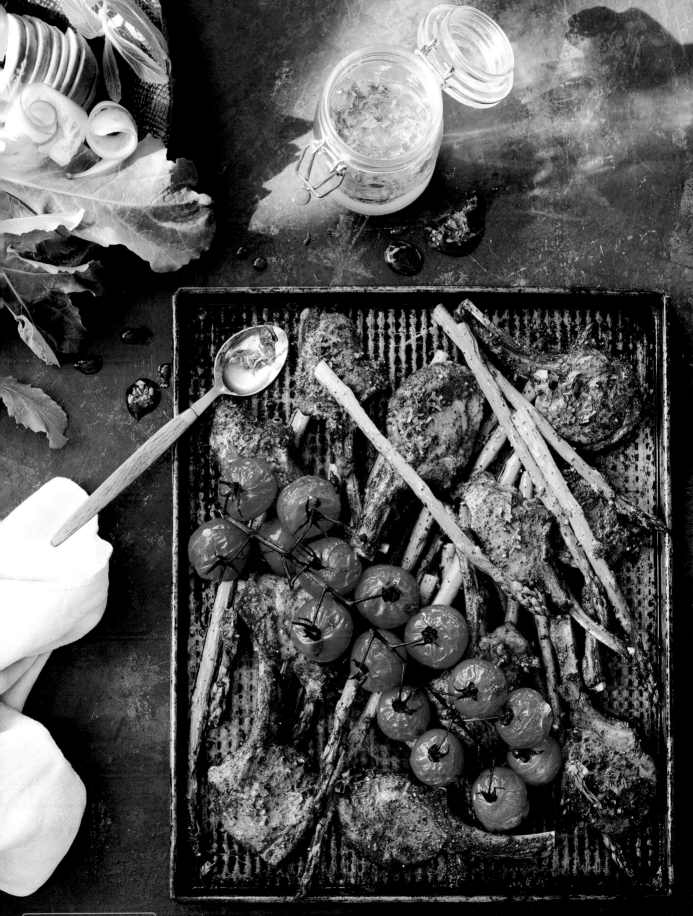

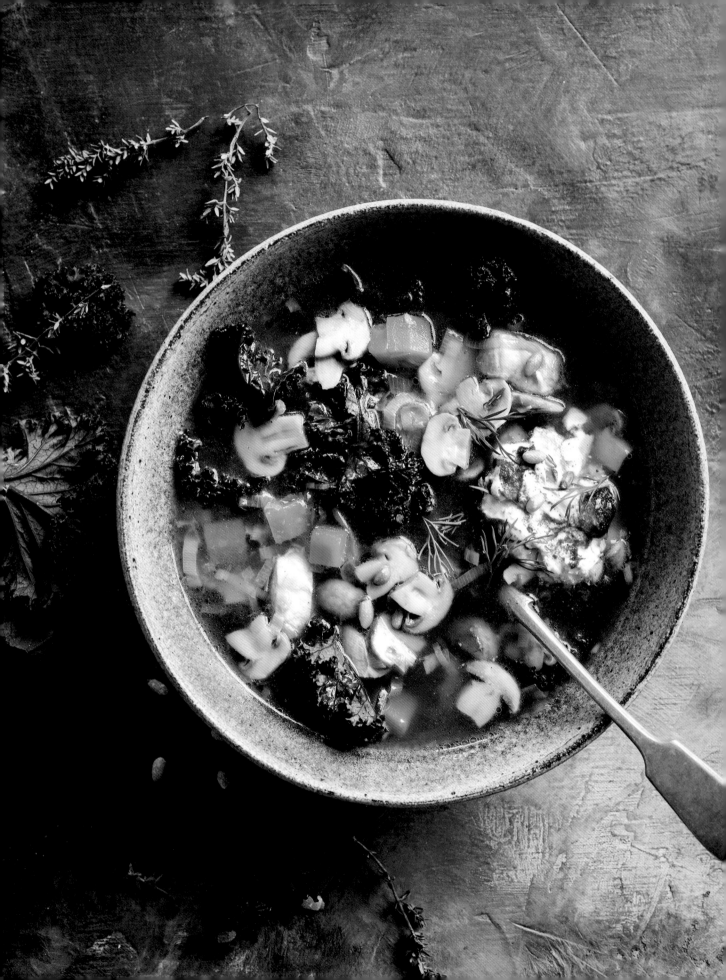

Chicken and mushroom soup with dill yoghurt

8 G CARB PER SERVE

🍴 **Serves 4**   🕐 **Preparation: 20–25 minutes**
🍲 **Cooking: 15 minutes**   ◎ **Difficulty: Easy**

1 tablespoon olive oil

600 g lean chicken
tenderloins, chopped

150 g leek, white part only, thinly sliced

150 g carrot, finely chopped

2 cloves garlic, crushed

500 g mixed mushrooms (button, field,
Swiss brown), sliced

3 sprigs thyme

1 litre salt-reduced vegetable stock

100 g kale leaves, torn into 3 cm pieces

80 g pine nuts, toasted

extra dill, to serve

DILL YOGHURT

100 g natural Greek-style yoghurt

¼ cup dill

2 teaspoons finely grated lemon zest

½ teaspoon sweet paprika

To make the dill yoghurt, combine all the ingredients in a small bowl. Season to taste with freshly ground black pepper. Chill until required.

Heat the olive oil in a large saucepan over high heat. Add the chicken, leek, carrot and crushed garlic and cook, stirring, for 3 minutes. Add the mushroom and thyme and cook, stirring, for 2 minutes.

Pour in the stock and cook, partially covered and stirring occasionally, for 10 minutes or until the vegetables are tender and the chicken is cooked through.

Remove the pan from the heat and stir through the kale until the leaves wilt. Season to taste with freshly ground black pepper.

Divide the soup among serving bowls. Serve topped with the dill yoghurt, pine nuts and extra dill.

> **WEEKS 7–12 CARB EXTRAS**
>
> For an extra 8 g carbs per serve, serve with 2 slices (½ slice per person) toasted mixed grain bread, or 1 slice toasted Herman Brot bread per person. (Herman Brot bread provides only 2.5 g carbs per serve, compared to 15 g carbs in a slice of regular bread.)

UNITS PER SERVE

Lean meat, fish, poultry, eggs, tofu: **1.5**
Low–moderate carb vegetables: **3**
Healthy fats: **2**

Lemongrass beef and broccolini stir-fry

6 G
CARB
PER
SERVE

🍴 **Serves 4**   🕐 **Preparation: 15–20 minutes**
🍳 **Cooking: 10 minutes**   ⏱ **Difficulty: Easy**

600 g lean beef rump steak,
  thinly sliced
2 stalks lemongrass, white part only,
  finely chopped
1 fresh long green chilli, finely chopped
4 cm piece ginger, finely grated
1 teaspoon ground white pepper
2 tablespoons rice bran oil
225 g seeded red capsicum, sliced
300 g broccolini, trimmed and cut into
  5 cm lengths
225 g baby pak choy, leaves separated
4 spring onions, thinly sliced diagonally
juice of 2 limes
75 g bean sprouts, trimmed

Combine the beef, lemongrass, chilli, ginger and white pepper in
a large bowl.

Heat the rice bran oil in a large wok over high heat. Add the beef
mixture in three batches and stir-fry for 2 minutes or until cooked
and golden. Transfer to a bowl.

Add the capsicum, broccolini, pak choy and ½ cup (125 ml) water
to the wok and stir-fry for 2 minutes or until the vegetables are just
tender. Return the beef and any juices to the wok and stir-fry for
1 minute.

Remove the wok from the heat and toss through the spring onion,
lime juice and bean sprouts. Serve.

WEEKS 7–12 CARB EXTRAS

For an extra 8–12 g carbs per serve, serve with 160 g (40 g per
person) cooked brown basmati rice or 200 g (50 g per person)
cooked quinoa.

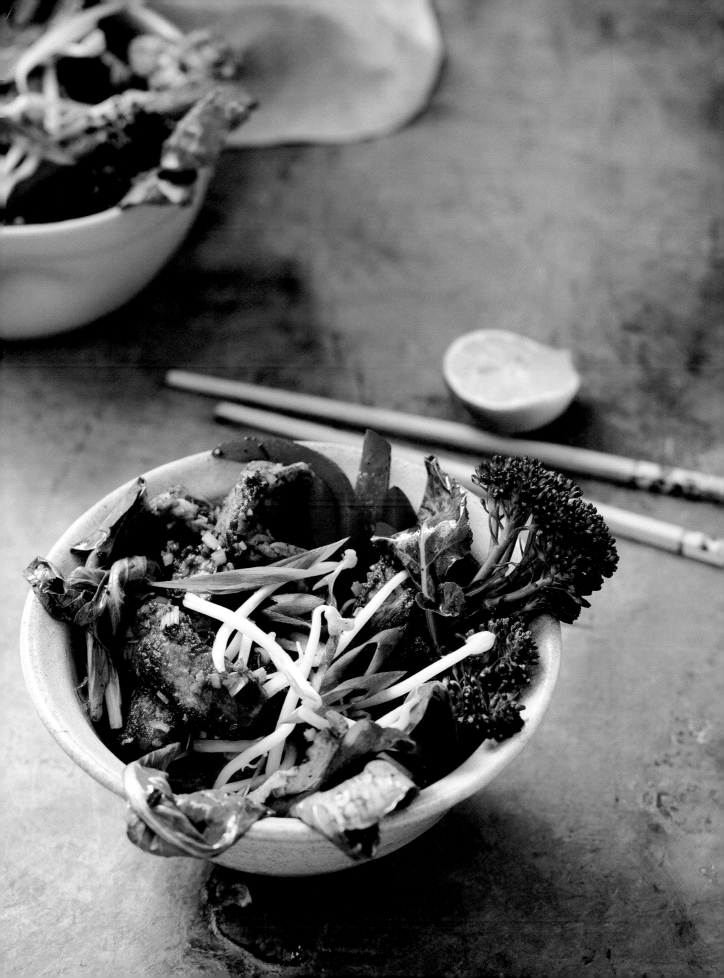

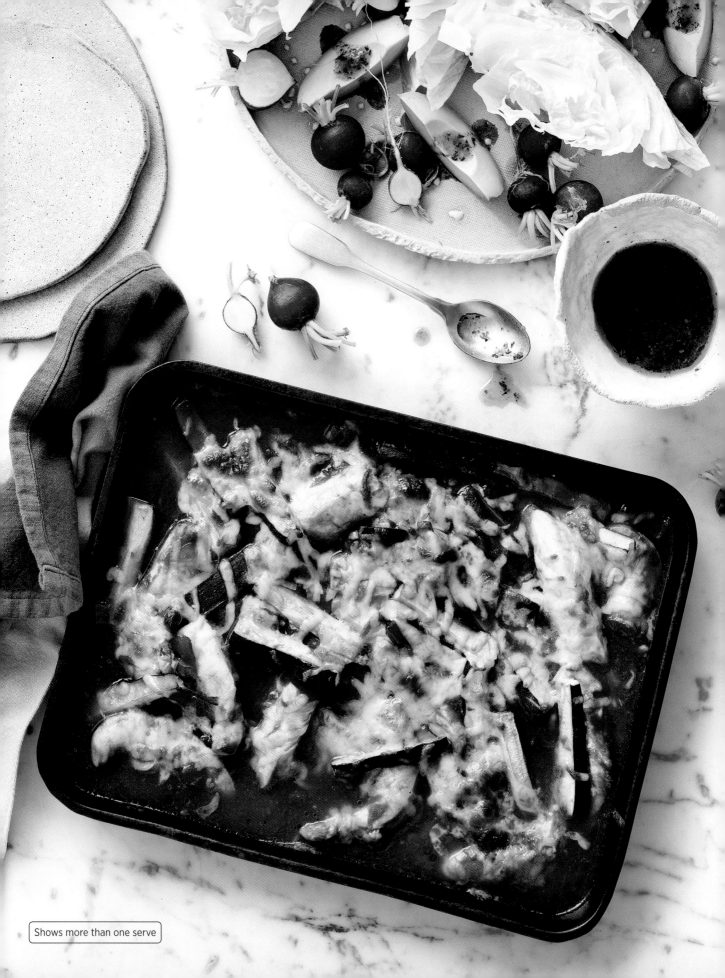

Shows more than one serve

Lean meat, fish, poultry, eggs, tofu: **1.5**
Dairy and dairy alternatives: **0.5**
Low–moderate carb vegetables: **2.5**
Healthy fats: **3**

300 g small iceberg lettuce,
  cut into wedges
150 g baby radishes, halved
160 g avocado, cut into wedges
finely grated zest and juice of 2 limes
2 teaspoons Mexican spice mix
1 tablespoon extra virgin olive oil

SALSA CHICKEN

1 x 300 g jar mild tomato salsa
600 g lean chicken tenderloins,
  halved lengthways
300 g zucchini, sliced into rounds
  or batons
1 cup (250 ml) salt-reduced
  chicken stock
50 g mozzarella, finely grated

Salsa chicken with avocado and radish salad

7 G
CARB
PER
SERVE

🍴 **Serves 4**   🕐 **Preparation: 15–20 minutes**
🍲 **Cooking: 15 minutes**   🌡 **Difficulty: Easy**

Preheat the oven to 220°C (200°C fan-forced). Place a baking dish in the oven to preheat.

To make the salsa chicken, combine the salsa, chicken, zucchini and stock in a large bowl. Season to taste with freshly ground black pepper. Carefully place the chicken mixture in the hot baking dish and sprinkle the mozzarella evenly over the top. Bake for 15 minutes or until the chicken is cooked and golden.

Meanwhile, divide the lettuce, radish and avocado among serving plates. Whisk together the lime zest and juice, spice mix and olive oil in a small jug and season to taste with freshly ground black pepper. Pour the dressing over the salads.

Divide the salsa chicken among the plates and serve.

WEEKS 7–12 CARB EXTRAS

For an extra 8 g carbs per serve, serve with 160 g (40 g per person) drained and rinsed tinned black beans or red kidney beans. Add to the plates with the lettuce, radish and avocado.

UNITS PER SERVE

Lean meat, fish, poultry, eggs, tofu: **1.5**
Dairy and dairy alternatives: **1.5**
Low-moderate carb vegetables: **3**
Healthy fats: **3**

1 tablespoon olive oil
600 g lean chicken tenderloins,
    finely chopped
1 clove garlic, crushed
1 tablespoon thyme leaves, plus
    2 teaspoons extra for sprinkling
300 g button mushrooms, halved
300 g yellow squash, sliced
    horizontally into rounds
8 eggs, lightly beaten
150 g haloumi, chopped

ALMOND TOMATOES

300 g cherry tomatoes, halved
2 tablespoons red wine vinegar
1 cup basil leaves
80 g whole natural almonds,
    toasted and chopped

Haloumi and chicken frittata with almond tomatoes

🍴 Serves 4   🕐 Preparation: 15–20 minutes
🍳 Cooking: 15 minutes   🎚 Difficulty: Easy

To make the almond tomatoes, mix together all the ingredients in a bowl and season to taste with freshly ground black pepper. Set aside until required.

Preheat the oven grill to high.

Heat the olive oil in a large heavy-based frying pan over high heat. Add the chicken, garlic, thyme, mushrooms and squash and cook, stirring occasionally, for 5 minutes or until the vegetables are starting to soften and the chicken is cooked.

Reduce the heat to medium. Add the egg. Cook, shaking the pan and stirring gently for 1 minute, then continue to cook untouched for 5 minutes or until the egg is set around the edges of the pan, but still wet in the centre. Sprinkle over the haloumi and extra thyme, then cook under the grill for 2–3 minutes or until set and golden.

Serve the frittata with the almond tomatoes.

> **WEEKS 7–12 CARB EXTRAS**
>
> For an extra 7–8 g carbs per serve, serve with 2 slices (½ slice per person) toasted mixed grain bread, or add 200 g (50 g per person) drained and rinsed tinned cannellini beans to the tomato mixture.

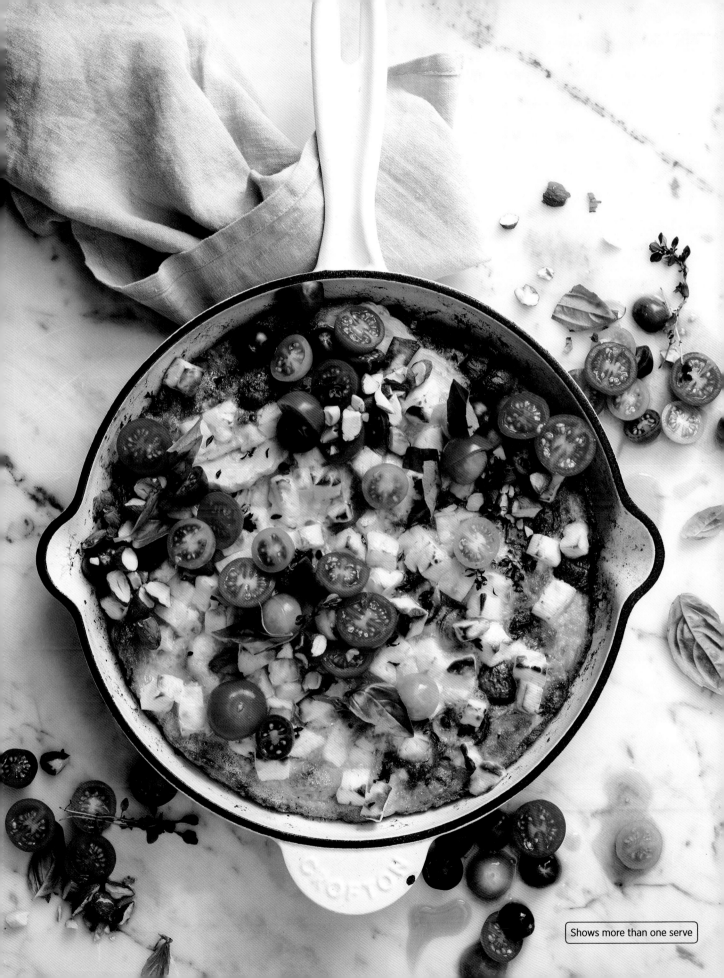

Shows more than one serve

UNITS PER SERVE
Lean meat, fish, poultry, eggs, tofu: **1.5**
Low–moderate carb vegetables: **4**
Healthy fats: **2**

Peppered pork and vegie smash

🍴 **Serves 4**   🕐 **Preparation: 15–20 minutes**
🍲 **Cooking: 10 minutes**   🎩 **Difficulty: Easy**

1 tablespoon olive oil
600 g lean pork tenderloin, sinew
   removed, thinly sliced diagonally
1 tablespoon freshly ground
   black pepper
1 cup small flat-leaf parsley leaves
½ cup oregano leaves
2 tablespoons chopped chives
finely grated zest and juice of 1 lemon
40 g pecans, toasted and chopped
25 g rocket leaves

VEGIE SMASH
300 g small broccoli florets
300 g zucchini, coarsely grated
300 g peeled celeriac, coarsely grated
1 cup (250 ml) salt-reduced
   chicken stock

To make the vegie smash, place all the ingredients in a saucepan over high heat and cook, stirring occasionally, for 10 minutes or until the vegetables are tender and the stock has reduced by two-thirds. Remove the pan from the heat. Smash everything together with a potato masher or fork and season to taste with freshly ground black pepper. Cover to keep warm.

Meanwhile, combine the olive oil, pork and pepper in a bowl. Heat a wok over high heat. Add the pork in three batches and stir-fry for 2 minutes each or until cooked and golden. Transfer to a bowl and cover to keep warm.

Combine the parsley, oregano, chives, lemon zest and juice, pecans and rocket in a large bowl.

Divide the vegie smash among serving plates and top with the pork. Serve with the parsley mixture.

WEEKS 7–12 CARB EXTRAS

For an extra 9 g carbs per serve, add 200 g (50 g per person) peeled and coarsely grated sweet potato to the vegie smash and cook as directed.

UNITS PER SERVE
Lean meat, fish, poultry, eggs, tofu: **1.5**
Dairy and dairy alternatives: **0.5**
Low–moderate carb vegetables: **3.5**
Healthy fats: **3**

Pesto tofu with raw vegetable noodles

11 G
CARB
PER
SERVE

🍴 **Serves 4**   🕐 **Preparation: 20–25 minutes**
🥘 **Cooking: 10 minutes**   👨‍🍳 **Difficulty: Easy**

1 tablespoon rice bran oil
600 g firm tofu, chopped
300 g tomatoes, finely chopped
300 g beetroot, spiralised into long
    thin noodles
300 g zucchini, spiralised into long
    thin noodles
small basil leaves, to garnish
lemon wedges, to serve

PESTO
2 teaspoons wholegrain mustard
2 cups basil leaves
1 clove garlic
80 g macadamias, toasted
40 g parmesan, finely grated
¼ cup (60 ml) red wine vinegar

To make the pesto, place all the ingredients in a small food processor and process until smooth and well combined, adding a little water if necessary to loosen. Set aside until required.

Heat the rice bran oil in a large frying pan over high heat. Add the tofu and cook, stirring, for 5 minutes or until crisp and golden. Add the tomato and cook, stirring, for 1 minute. Add the pesto and ½ cup (125 ml) water, then remove the pan from the heat and stir until the mixture is well combined. Season to taste with freshly ground black pepper.

Divide the beetroot and zucchini noodles among plates and top with the pesto and tofu mixture. Garnish with basil leaves and serve lemon wedges alongside.

WEEKS 7–12 CARB EXTRAS

For an extra 7 g carbs per serve, serve with 200 g (50 g per person) drained and rinsed tinned cannellini beans.

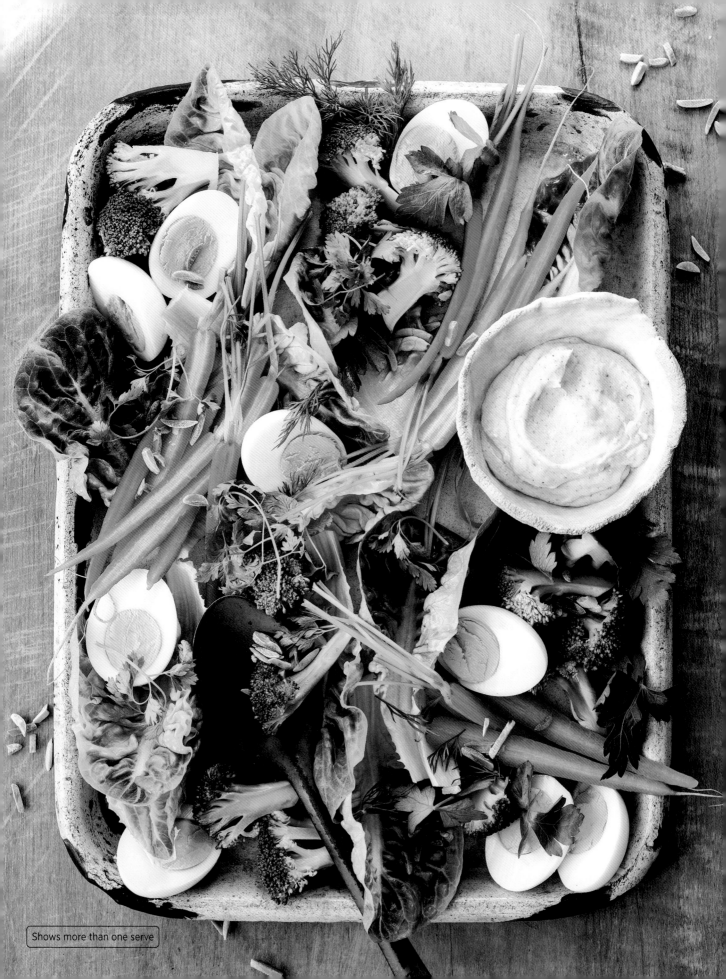

Shows more than one serve

Egg salad with avocado dressing

UNITS PER SERVE
Lean meat, fish, poultry, eggs, tofu: **1.5**
Dairy and dairy alternatives: **0.5**
Low–moderate carb vegetables: **3.5**
Healthy fats: **3**

Serves 4 **Preparation: 15–20 minutes**
Cooking: 10 minutes **Difficulty: Easy**

8 eggs
300 g broccoli florets
300 g baby carrots, trimmed and
   scrubbed, halved lengthways
300 g baby cos lettuce,
   leaves separated
1 cup flat-leaf parsley leaves
½ cup chervil leaves or chopped chives
¼ cup dill
40 g slivered almonds, toasted

AVOCADO DRESSING
160 g avocado
110 g cottage cheese
finely grated zest and juice of 1 lemon
2 teaspoons sumac (see note)

To make the avocado dressing, process all the ingredients in a small food processor until smooth and well combined. Season to taste with freshly ground black pepper. Set aside until required.

Meanwhile, boil the eggs in a saucepan of boiling water for 5 minutes. Add the broccoli and carrot to the same pan and cook for 1 minute. Drain. Carefully peel the eggs while they are still warm, then halve lengthways.

Combine the cos, parsley, chervil and dill in a bowl, then divide among serving plates. Top with the egg halves and vegetables and sprinkle with the slivered almonds. Serve with the avocado dressing.

WEEKS 7–12 CARB EXTRAS

For an extra 9 g carbs per serve, add 160 g (40 g per person) drained and rinsed tinned lentils to the cos mixture.

Note: You can swap the sumac for sweet paprika, if desired.

UNITS PER SERVE
Lean meat, fish, poultry, eggs, tofu: **1.5**
Dairy and dairy alternatives: **0.5**
Low–moderate carb vegetables: **4**
Healthy fats: **3**

Chicken curry with cucumber yoghurt salad

14 G CARB PER SERVE

🍴 **Serves 4**   🕐 **Preparation: 20–25 minutes**
🍲 **Cooking: 15 minutes**   🎖 **Difficulty: Easy**

1 tablespoon olive oil
600 g lean chicken breast fillets,
    cut into 2 cm pieces
1 tablespoon curry powder
1 cup (250 ml) tomato passata
2 cups (500 ml) salt-reduced
    chicken stock
300 g carrots, halved lengthways,
    diagonally sliced
250 g eggplant, cut into 2 cm pieces
extra coriander sprigs, to serve

CUCUMBER YOGHURT SALAD

200 g low-fat natural
    Greek-style yoghurt
¼ cup chopped mint
finely grated zest and juice of 1 lemon
300 g Lebanese cucumber, halved
    lengthways, sliced diagonally
50 g baby spinach leaves
½ cup small coriander sprigs
80 g blanched almonds, toasted
    and chopped

Heat the olive oil in a large saucepan over high heat. Add the chicken and curry powder and cook, stirring, for 3 minutes. Add the passata, stock, carrot and eggplant, then cover and cook, stirring occasionally, for 10 minutes or until the chicken and vegetables are cooked and the sauce has reduced slightly.

Meanwhile, to make the cucumber yoghurt salad, combine the yoghurt, mint, lemon zest and juice in a small bowl. Season to taste with freshly ground black pepper. Arrange the cucumber, spinach, coriander and almonds in a serving dish, with the bowl of yoghurt dressing alongside. Garnish with extra coriander.

Divide the chicken curry among bowls and serve with the cucumber yoghurt salad.

> **WEEKS 7–12 CARB EXTRAS**
>
> For an extra 8 g carbs per serve, serve with 200 g (50 g per person) cooked quinoa.

Note: Depending on your brand of yoghurt you may find the dressing is a little thick. If so, just add 1–2 tablespoons water to thin it down to a runny consistency.

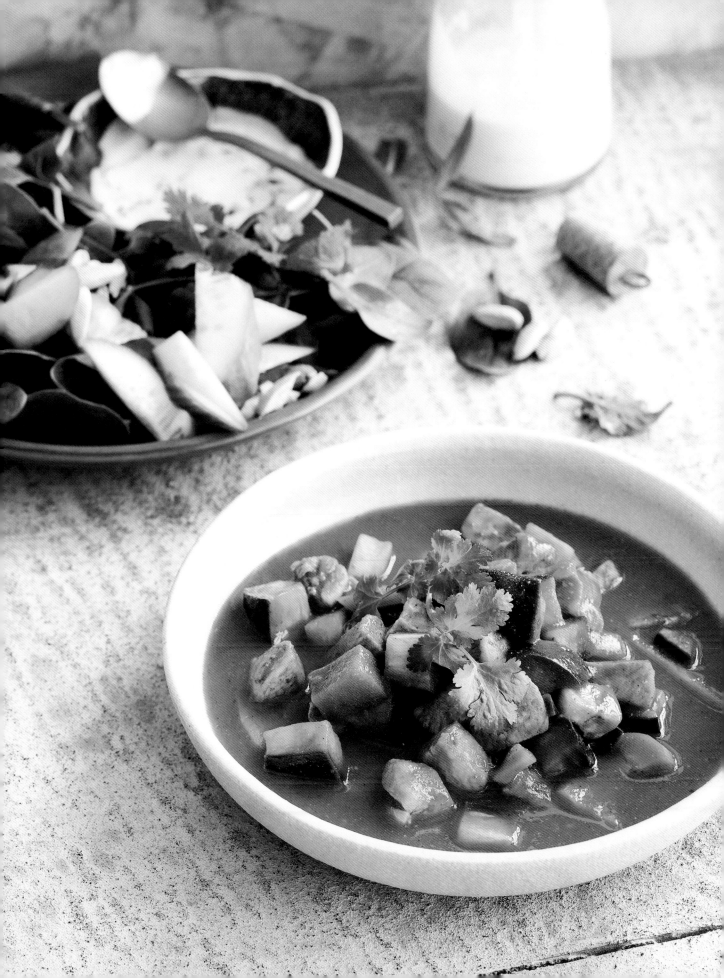

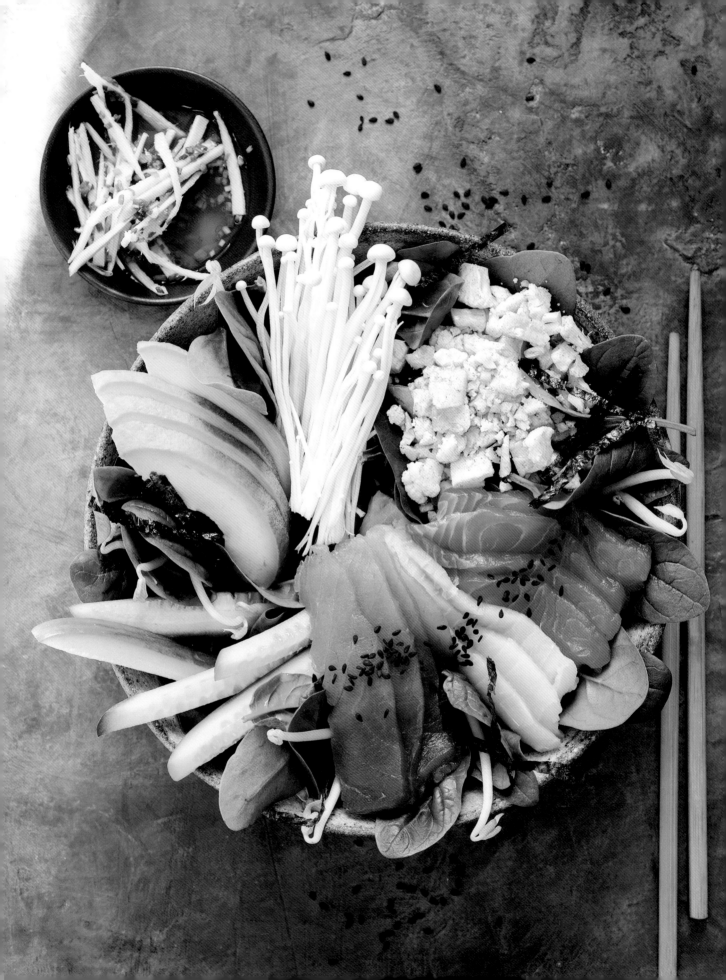

UNITS PER SERVE
Lean meat, fish, poultry, eggs, tofu: **1.5**
Low–moderate carb vegetables: **3**
Healthy fats: **5**

Raw sushi bowls with pickled ginger

5 G CARB PER SERVE

🍴 **Serves 4**   🕐 **Preparation: 15–20 minutes, plus standing time**
🍲 **Cooking: Nil**   🍳 **Difficulty: Easy**

75 g baby spinach leaves
150 g bean sprouts, trimmed
1 sheet nori, shredded
300 g cauliflower florets
1 teaspoon ground turmeric
600 g mixed, very thinly sliced
   sashimi (tuna, salmon, swordfish)
300 g Lebanese cucumber,
   cut into batons
75 g enoki mushrooms
240 g avocado, sliced
2 tablespoons black sesame seeds
   (see note)

PICKLED GINGER

5 cm piece ginger, peeled,
   cut into long thin strips
¼ cup (60 ml) apple cider vinegar
1 tablespoon chopped chives

To make the pickled ginger, combine all the ingredients in a small bowl. Stand at room temperature for 20 minutes.

Combine the baby spinach, bean sprouts and nori in a bowl, then divide among four serving bowls.

Place the cauliflower and turmeric in a food processor and process for 20 seconds or until some of the cauliflower resembles rice grains. Divide among the serving bowls.

Add the sashimi, cucumber, mushrooms and avocado to the serving bowls and sprinkle with the sesame seeds. Serve with the pickled ginger.

WEEKS 7–12 CARB EXTRAS

For an extra 7 g carbs per serve, add 160 g (40 g per person) corn kernels to the bowls.

Note: You can buy black sesame seeds from the spice section in greengrocers or Asian supermarkets. If you can't find them, use toasted white sesame seeds instead.

Lean meat, fish, poultry, eggs, tofu: **1.5**
Low–moderate carb vegetables: **4**
Healthy fats: **4**

Seafood tagine with almond broccoli couscous

10 G CARB PER SERVE

1 tablespoon olive oil
300 g fennel, thinly sliced lengthways
300 g peeled celeriac, cut into
 thick matchsticks
1 tablespoon salt-reduced tomato paste
large pinch saffron threads
3 teaspoons ground cumin
3 teaspoons ground coriander
600 g fresh marinara mix (fish, prawns,
 calamari, octopus, mussels)
2 cups (500 ml) salt-reduced fish stock
1 cup coriander sprigs,
 plus extra to serve
lemon wedges, to serve

ALMOND BROCCOLI COUSCOUS

120 g whole natural almonds, toasted
300 g broccoli florets
½ cup chopped flat-leaf parsley

🍴 **Serves 4** 🕒 **Preparation: 15–20 minutes**
🎛 **Cooking: 15 minutes** ✋ **Difficulty: Easy**

To make the almond broccoli couscous, process the almonds in a food processor until finely chopped. Add the broccoli and parsley and process for 20 seconds or until finely chopped. Season to taste with freshly ground black pepper. Set aside.

Heat the olive oil in a large deep frying pan over high heat. Add the fennel and celeriac and cook, stirring, for 3 minutes or until starting to soften. Add the tomato paste, saffron, cumin and coriander and cook, stirring, for 1 minute or until fragrant.

Add the marinara mix and stock and cook, covered and shaking the pan occasionally, for 10 minutes or until the seafood is just cooked and the stock has reduced by half. Remove the pan from the heat and stir the coriander through.

Divide the seafood tagine among shallow serving bowls. Spoon the almond broccoli couscous on top and serve with extra coriander.

WEEKS 7–12 CARB EXTRAS

For an extra 9 g carbs per serve, add 200 g (50 g per person) peeled and grated sweet potato to the fennel mixture when cooking.

Note: If you have one, use a mandoline to slice your cucumber and radishes very thinly.

You can use 300 g thickly sliced celery or zucchini in place of the celeriac, if preferred.

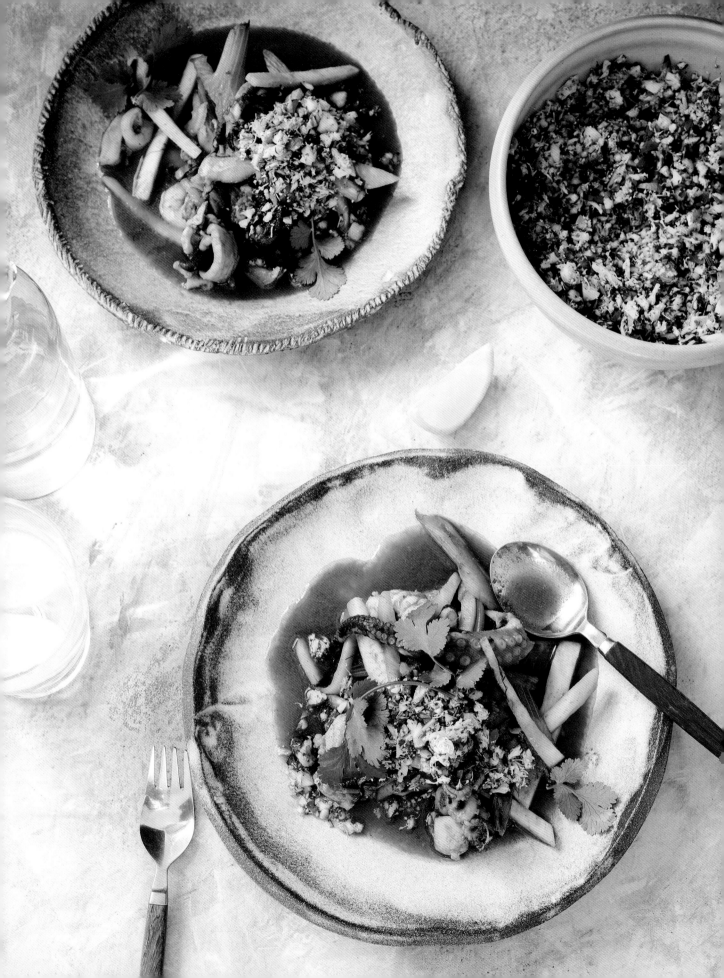

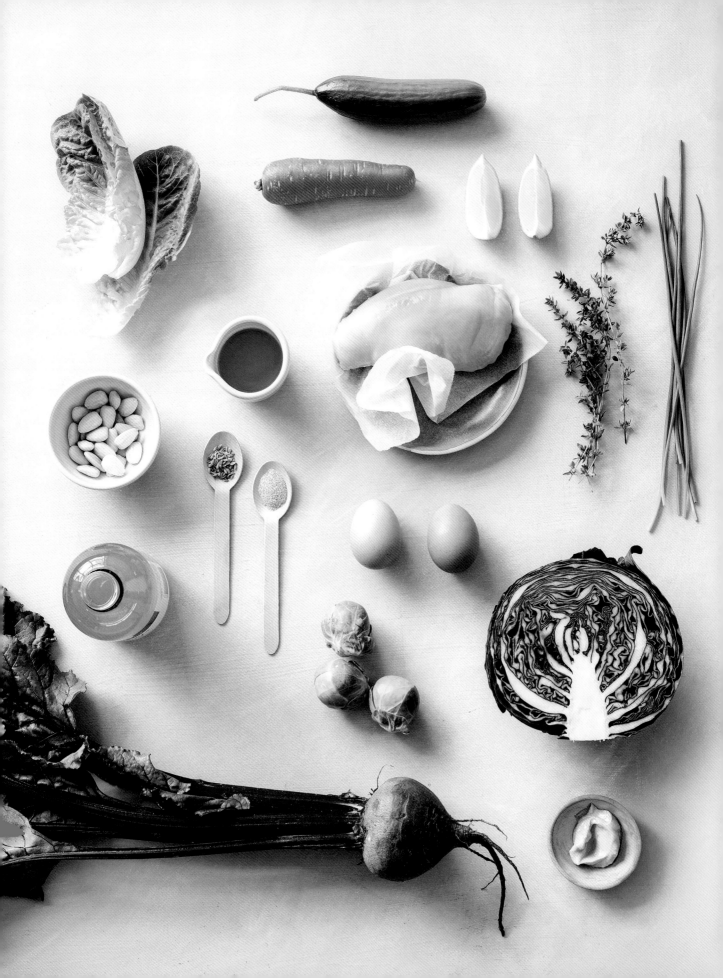

Crunchy chicken and rainbow salad

UNITS PER SERVE
Lean meat, fish, poultry, eggs, tofu: **1.5**
Low–moderate carb vegetables: **3**
Healthy fats: **4**

🍽 Serves 4 　 🕐 Preparation: 25–30 minutes
🍲 Cooking: 15 minutes 　 🥄 Difficulty: Easy

2 eggs
500 g lean chicken breast fillets,
　 thinly sliced
80 g blanched almonds,
　 very finely chopped
2 tablespoons finely chopped tarragon
2 tablespoons thyme leaves
2 tablespoons chopped chives
1 teaspoon garlic powder
2 tablespoons olive oil
150 g baby cos lettuce,
　 leaves separated
lemon wedges, to serve

RAINBOW SALAD

2 teaspoons Dijon mustard
2 teaspoons fennel seeds
⅓ cup (80 ml) apple cider vinegar
150 g red cabbage, very finely shredded
100 g carrot, coarsely grated
50 g peeled beetroot, coarsely grated
150 g brussels sprouts,
　 very finely shredded
300 g Lebanese cucumbers,
　 cut into matchsticks

To make the rainbow salad, mix together the mustard, fennel seeds and vinegar in a large bowl. Season to taste with freshly ground black pepper. Add the remaining salad ingredients and toss until well combined. Chill until required.

Lightly beat the eggs in a large bowl. Add the chicken, almonds, tarragon, thyme, chives and garlic powder, and season to taste with freshly ground black pepper. Toss until everything is well combined and the chicken is evenly coated.

Heat the olive oil in a large frying pan over medium–high heat. Add the chicken in two batches and cook, turning occasionally, for 7 minutes or until golden and cooked through. Transfer to a plate and cover to keep warm.

Divide the cos leaves and rainbow salad among serving plates or bowls. Top with the chicken and serve with lemon wedges.

WEEKS 7–12 CARB EXTRAS

For an extra 8 g carbs per serve, serve with 200 g (50 g per person) cooked quinoa.

Shows more than one serve

UNITS PER SERVE
Lean meat, fish, poultry, eggs, tofu: **1.5**
Low–moderate carb vegetables: **3**
Healthy fats: **2**

Seared tuna with tomato beans and fried capers

6 G
CARB
PER
SERVE

🍴 **Serves 4**   🕐 **Preparation: 15–20 minutes**
🍳 **Cooking: 10 minutes**   👨‍🍳 **Difficulty: Easy**

300 g green beans, trimmed
300 g tomatoes, finely chopped
2 cloves garlic, crushed
1 cup (250 ml) salt-reduced
    chicken stock
2 tablespoons extra virgin olive oil
2 tablespoons capers in brine,
    rinsed and patted dry
4 x 150 g tuna steaks
150 g asparagus, trimmed and
    halved crossways
50 g rocket leaves
150 g Lebanese cucumber, cut
    with a vegetable peeler into long
    thin ribbons
finely grated zest and juice of 1 lemon

Combine the beans, tomato, garlic and stock in a saucepan over medium–high heat. Cook, stirring occasionally, for 10 minutes or until the beans are very tender and the stock has reduced by half. Season to taste with freshly ground black pepper.

Meanwhile, heat the olive oil in a large frying pan over high heat. Add the capers and cook, stirring, for 2 minutes or until crispy. Pour the mixture into a heatproof jug and set aside until required.

Season the tuna on all sides with freshly ground black pepper. Add the tuna and asparagus to the frying pan and cook, turning the tuna once, for 4 minutes for medium or until cooked to your liking and the asparagus is tender. Transfer to a plate and cover to keep warm.

Combine the rocket, cucumber, lemon zest and juice in a large bowl and season to taste with freshly ground black pepper. Divide among serving plates. Add the bean mixture and top with the tuna and asparagus. Spoon the caper oil over and serve.

WEEKS 7–12 CARB EXTRAS

For an extra 9 g carbs per serve, add 200 g (50 g per person) peeled and finely chopped sweet potato to the bean mixture during cooking.

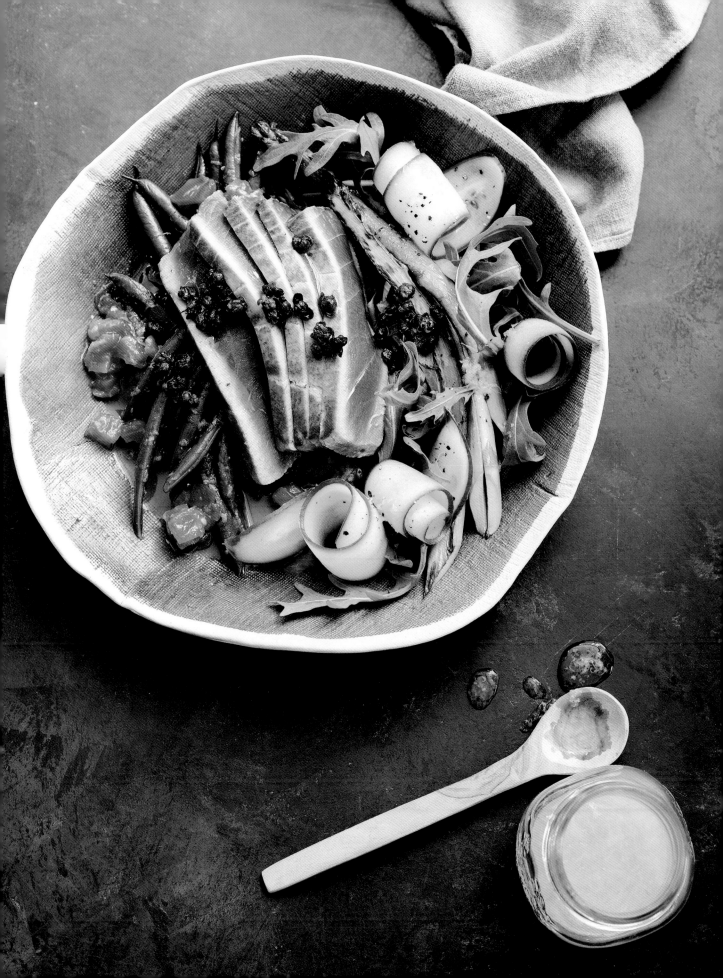

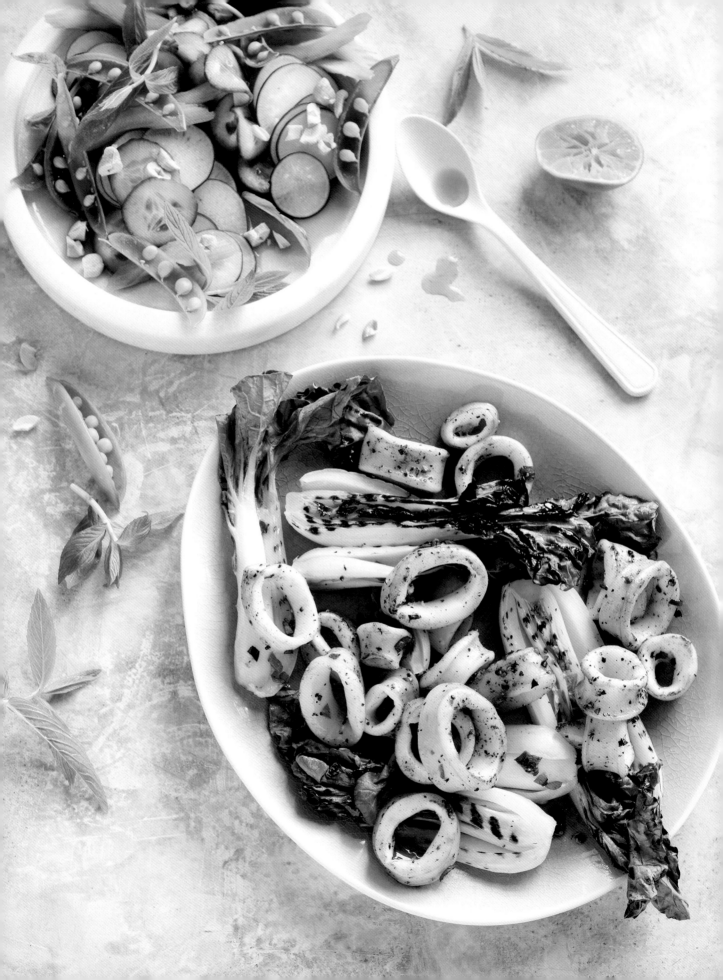

UNITS PER SERVE

Lean meat, fish, poultry, eggs, tofu: **1.5**

Low-moderate carb vegetables: **3.5**

Healthy fats: **3**

Chilli calamari with cucumber, cashew and mint salad

🍴 Serves 4   🕐 Preparation: 20–25 minutes, plus standing time

🍲 Cooking: 5 minutes   🎩 Difficulty: Easy

600 g small cleaned calamari hoods,
   cut into rings
1 tablespoon olive oil
1 fresh long red chilli, finely chopped
2 teaspoons freshly ground
   black pepper
300 g baby pak choy,
   halved lengthways
1 lime, cut into thick wedges

CUCUMBER, CASHEW AND MINT SALAD

300 g Lebanese cucumber, very thinly
   sliced into rounds (see note)
1 tablespoon white wine vinegar
1 tablespoon salt-reduced soy sauce
75 g celery stalks, thinly
   sliced diagonally
75 g radishes, very thinly sliced
   into rounds
150 g sugar snap peas, trimmed
   and halved lengthways
1 cup small mint leaves
80 g cashews, toasted and chopped

Heat a barbecue flat plate and chargrill to high.

To make the cucumber, cashew and mint salad, combine the cucumber, vinegar and soy sauce in a bowl. Leave to stand, tossing occasionally, for 5 minutes or until the cucumber has softened. Add the remaining ingredients and gently toss to combine. Set aside.

Combine the calamari, olive oil, chilli and pepper in a bowl. Cook on the barbecue flat plate, turning occasionally, for 2–3 minutes or until just tender and golden. At the same time, cook the pak choy on the chargrill for 2–3 minutes.

Serve the calamari and vegetables with the cucumber, cashew and mint salad and lime wedges.

WEEKS 7–12 CARB EXTRAS

For an extra 8 g carbs per serve, serve with 200 g (50 g per person) cooked quinoa.

Note: If you have one, use a mandoline to slice your cucumber and radishes very thinly.

Tofu with five spice mushrooms and coriander salsa

🍽 **Serves 4**   🕐 **Preparation: 20–25 minutes**

🍳 **Cooking: 5 minutes**   👩‍🍳 **Difficulty: Easy**

2 tablespoons Shaoxing rice wine
  or dry sherry

1 teaspoon sesame oil

3 cm piece ginger, finely grated

¼ teaspoon Chinese five spice

600 g mixed mushrooms, trimmed

600 g firm tofu, cut into 4 cm pieces

75 g bean sprouts, trimmed

CORIANDER SALSA

1 cup coriander leaves

2 spring onions, thinly sliced

75 g green beans, trimmed and thinly
  sliced into rounds

80 g firm avocado, finely chopped

finely grated zest and juice of 2 limes

Heat a barbecue flat plate to medium–high.

Combine the rice wine, sesame oil, ginger and five spice in a large bowl. Set aside until required.

Cook the mushrooms and tofu on the barbecue flat plate, turning occasionally, for 5 minutes or until cooked and golden on all sides. Immediately transfer to the five spice mixture in the bowl. Add the bean sprouts and toss gently to combine. Season to taste with freshly ground black pepper.

Meanwhile, to make the coriander salsa, mix together all the ingredients in a bowl, then season to taste with freshly ground black pepper.

Divide the mushrooms and tofu among serving plates. Top with the coriander salsa and serve.

WEEKS 7–12 CARB EXTRAS

For an extra 9 g carbs per serve, add 200 g (50 g per person) very thin slices of unpeeled sweet potato to the chargrill when cooking the tofu.

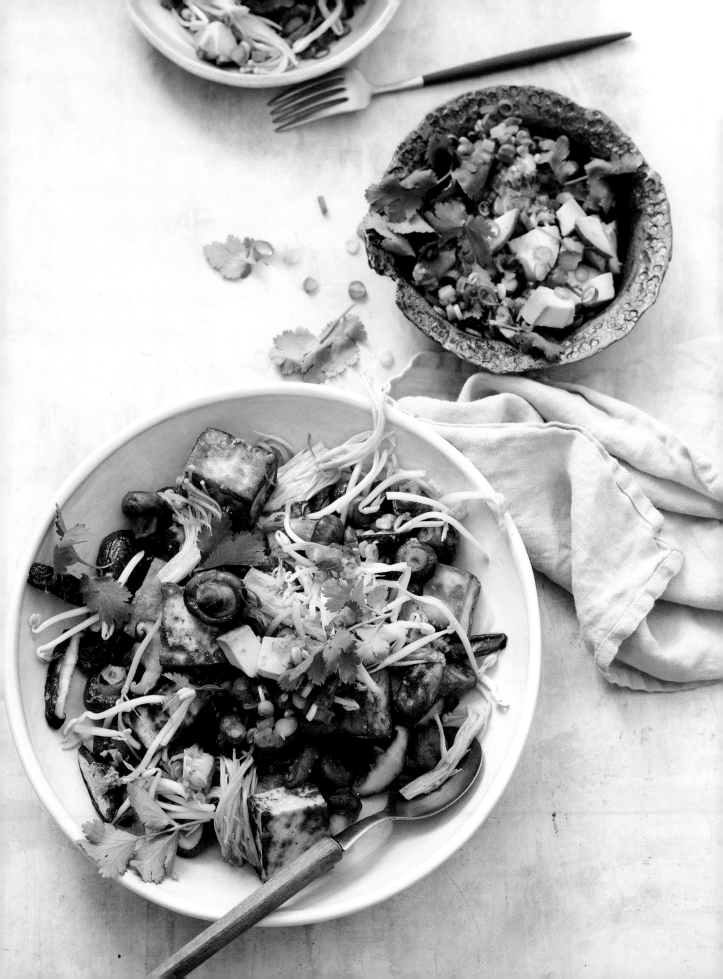

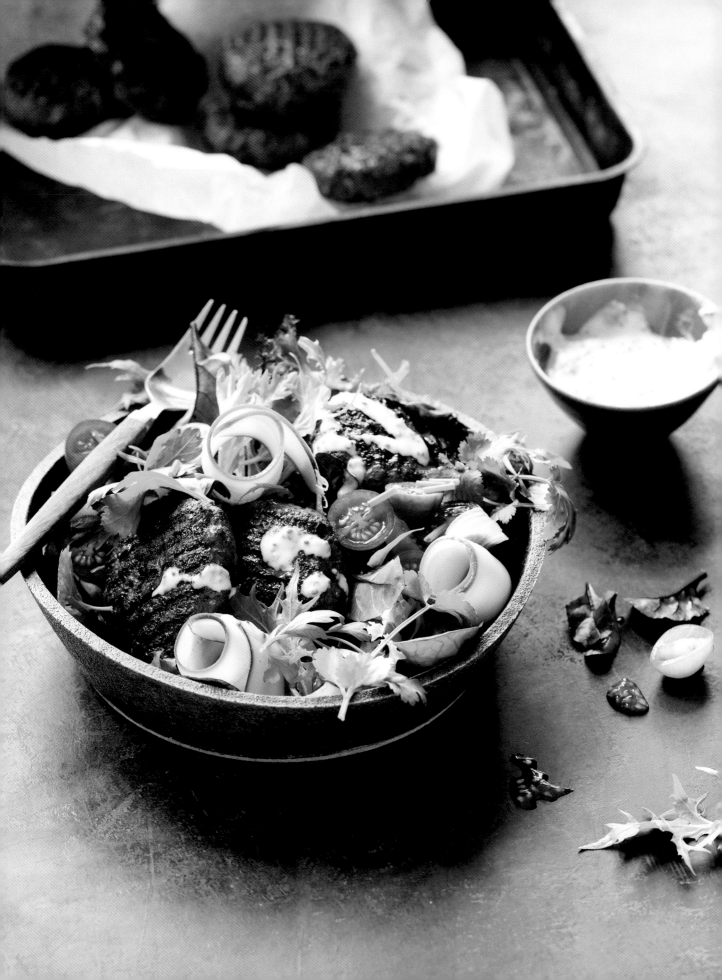

UNITS PER SERVE
Lean meat, fish, poultry, eggs, tofu: **1.5**
Low–moderate carb vegetables: **2.5**
Healthy fats: **2**

Beetroot and beef rissoles with herb salad and mustard tahini

🍴 **Serves 4** 🕐 **Preparation: 25–30 minutes**
🍳 **Cooking: 10 minutes** 👁 **Difficulty: Easy**

75 g mixed salad leaves
1 cup mixed herbs (flat-leaf parsley,
  basil, chives, tarragon)
300 g cherry tomatoes,
  halved or quartered
150 g zucchini, cut with a vegetable
  peeler into long thin ribbons
finely grated zest and juice of 1 lemon

MUSTARD TAHINI

2 tablespoons tahini
3 teaspoons wholegrain mustard
finely grated zest and juice of 1 lemon

RISSOLES

600 g lean beef, chopped
1 egg
150 g beetroot, skin scrubbed,
  coarsely grated
150 g carrot, coarsely grated
1 clove garlic, crushed

To make the mustard tahini, mix together all the ingredients with 2–3 tablespoons warm water in a small bowl (the mixture will be quite thick). Season to taste with freshly ground black pepper. Set aside until required. You may want to add a little extra warm water before serving if it has thickened further on standing.

To make the rissoles, place all the ingredients in a food processor and process until minced. Using slightly damp hands, divide the mixture into 12 equal portions and roll into rissoles.

Heat a barbecue chargrill to medium. Cook the rissoles for 4–5 minutes each side or until golden and cooked through.

Meanwhile, toss together the salad leaves, mixed herbs, tomato, zucchini, lemon zest and juice in a large bowl. Season to taste with freshly ground black pepper. Divide among serving bowls.

Divide the rissoles among the bowls. Spoon over the mustard tahini and serve.

WEEKS 7–12 CARB EXTRAS

For an extra 8 g carbs per serve, add 200 g (50 g per person) cooked quinoa to the salad.

UNITS PER SERVE

Lean meat, fish, poultry, eggs, tofu: **1.5**
Dairy and dairy alternatives: **1**
Low–moderate carb vegetables: **3**
Healthy fats: **1**

Chicken and vegetable stacks with haloumi

9 G CARB PER SERVE

🍴 **Serves 4**   🕐 **Preparation: 20–25 minutes**
🍳 **Cooking: 15 minutes**   🎖 **Difficulty: Easy**

300 g small yellow squash, halved
300 g broccolini, trimmed and
    halved lengthways
1 red onion (150 g), thinly sliced
    into rounds
3 x 200 g lean chicken breast fillets,
    each cut horizontally into 4 thin slices
1 tablespoon sweet paprika
100 g haloumi, chopped
basil leaves, to serve

PECAN PESTO

40 g pecans, toasted
2 cups basil leaves
1 fresh long green chilli, halved
    lengthways, seeded
finely grated zest and juice of 2 limes

Heat a barbecue flat plate and chargrill to medium–high.

To make the pecan pesto, place all the ingredients in a small food processor and process until smooth and well combined. Season to taste with freshly ground black pepper. Set aside until required.

Cook the squash, broccolini and onion on the flat plate, turning occasionally, for 5 minutes or until just cooked and golden. Transfer to a plate and cover to keep warm.

Meanwhile, sprinkle both sides of the chicken pieces with the sweet paprika and season to taste with freshly ground black pepper. Cook the chicken on the chargrill, turning occasionally, for 5 minutes or until golden and cooked through. Transfer to a heatproof plate and cover to keep warm.

Add the haloumi to the flat plate and cook, tossing, for 1 minute or until softened and golden.

Evenly stack the chicken and vegetables on serving plates and scatter over the haloumi. Dollop with the pecan pesto. Scatter over the basil leaves, season to taste with freshly ground black pepper and serve.

WEEKS 7–12 CARB EXTRAS

For an extra 6 g carbs per serve, heat 160 g (40 g per person) drained and rinsed tinned chickpeas on the barbecue flat plate for 1 minute and serve with the chicken and vegetable stacks.

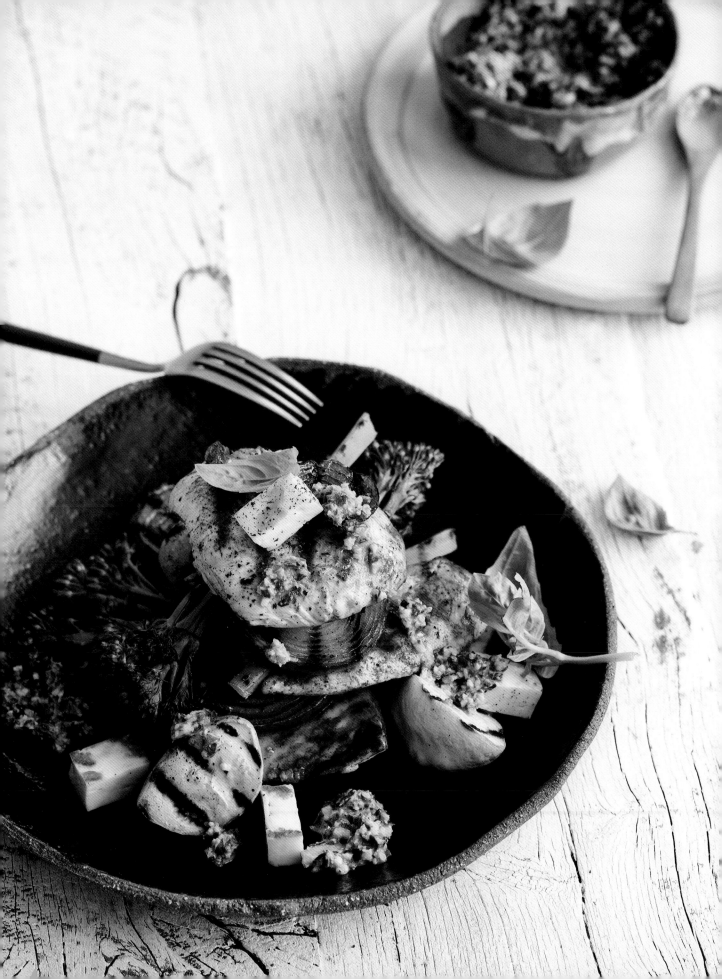

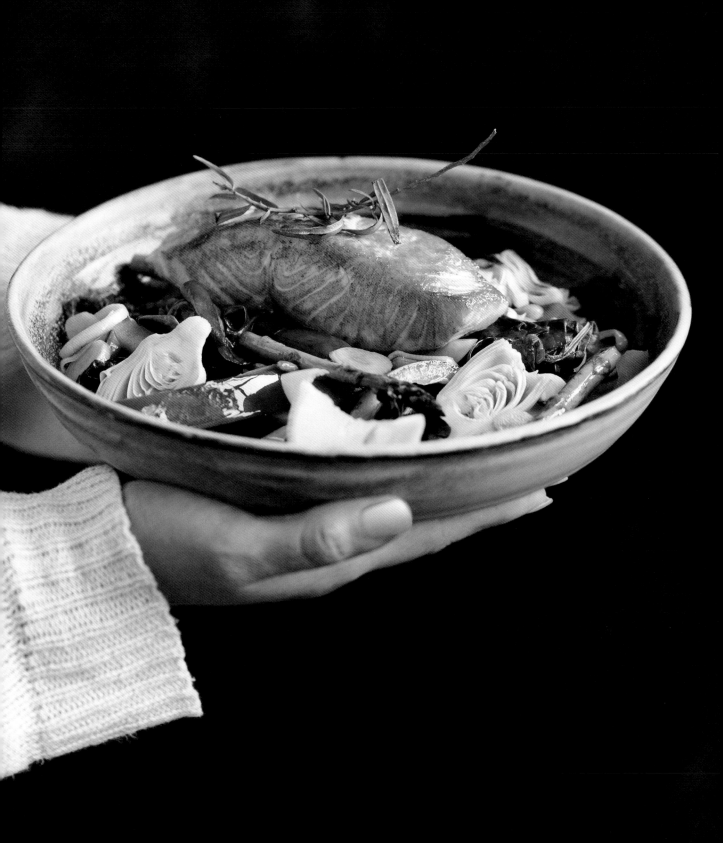

UNITS PER SERVE

Lean meat, fish, poultry, eggs, tofu: **1.5**

Low-moderate carb vegetables: **2.5**

Healthy fats: **1**

Salmon with Mediterranean vegetables

🍴 **Serves 4**   🕐 **Preparation: 15–20 minutes**
🍳 **Cooking: 10 minutes**   👨‍🍳 **Difficulty: Easy**

75 g leek, white part only, thinly sliced into rounds

225 g mixed capsicums (red, green, yellow), seeded and thinly sliced

2 cloves garlic, sliced

150 g asparagus, trimmed and halved crossways

75 g drained artichoke hearts in brine, halved

1 tablespoon capers in brine, rinsed

150 g baby spinach leaves

2 tablespoons tarragon leaves, plus extra to serve

40 g pine nuts, toasted

4 x 150 g salmon fillets, skin removed and pin-boned

lemon wedges, to serve

Heat a barbecue flat plate to medium–high.

Place the leek, capsicum and garlic on the flat plate and cook for 3 minutes, tossing occasionally. Add the asparagus, artichoke and capers and cook, tossing, for 1 minute or until all the vegetables are softened and light golden. Transfer to a large bowl. Season to taste with freshly ground black pepper.

Add the baby spinach to the flat plate in batches and cook for 30 seconds each or until just starting to wilt and soften. Transfer to the bowl with the other vegetables. Season to taste with freshly ground black pepper. Add the tarragon and pine nuts and toss together until well combined. Cover to keep warm.

Season the salmon fillets with freshly ground black pepper on both sides. Cook on the flat plate for 2–3 minutes each side for medium, or until cooked to your liking.

Serve the salmon with the Mediterranean vegetables and lemon wedges, topped with extra tarragon.

> **WEEKS 7–12 CARB EXTRAS**
>
> For an extra 9 g carbs per serve, serve with 200 g (50 g per person) thinly sliced, chargrilled sweet potato rounds.

UNITS PER SERVE

Lean meat, fish, poultry, eggs, tofu: **1.5**
Low–moderate carb vegetables: **3**
Healthy fats: **2**

Ginger and lime fish cakes with soy chargrilled veg

3 G
CARB
PER
SERVE

🍴 Serves 4   🕐 Preparation: 25–30 minutes, plus refrigerating time
🍲 Cooking: 15 minutes   🥄 Difficulty: Easy

150 g sugar snap peas
300 g broccoli florets
150 g Chinese broccoli, trimmed
   and cut into 7 cm lengths
160 g avocado, sliced
2 tablespoons salt-reduced soy sauce
lime wedges, to serve

PATTIES

550 g red fish fillets, skin removed,
   pin-boned
1 egg
75 g cooked and cooled Jerusalem
   artichoke (see notes)
1 small fresh red chilli
2 cm piece ginger, chopped
2 kaffir lime leaves, very
   thinly shredded
75 g green beans, trimmed and
   very thinly sliced into rounds

To make the patties, place the fish, egg, artichoke, chilli, ginger and kaffir lime leaves in a food processor and process until smooth and well combined, with a sticky texture. Stir through the green beans and season to taste with freshly ground black pepper. With slightly damp hands, divide the mixture into 12 even portions and shape into flat patties. Place on a baking tray lined with baking paper and chill for at least 20 minutes to set firm.

Heat a barbecue flat plate and chargrill to medium–high.

Cook the patties on the flat plate for 4 minutes each side or until cooked through and golden. Transfer to a plate and cover to keep warm.

Add the sugar snap peas, broccoli and Chinese broccoli to the chargrill and cook, turning occasionally, for 5 minutes or until just tender and golden. Transfer to a large bowl. Add the avocado and soy sauce and season to taste with freshly ground black pepper. Toss very gently to combine.

Serve the fish cakes with the vegetable mixture and lime wedges.

> **WEEKS 7–12 CARB EXTRAS**
>
> For an extra 8 g carbs per serve, serve with 200 g (50 g per person) cooked quinoa.

Notes: To cook Jerusalem artichoke, cut it into 2 cm pieces and place in a microwave-safe bowl with a splash of water. Cover and microwave on high for 6–8 minutes. Drain well, then allow to cool before using in the recipe. You can also steam the Jerusalem artichoke for 10–12 minutes. Do not boil it as this will make the mixture too wet.

If you can't find Jerusalem artichoke, simply replace it with the same quantity of peeled celeriac and cook as directed.

You could use the same amount of skinned, boned salmon in place of red fish, if preferred.

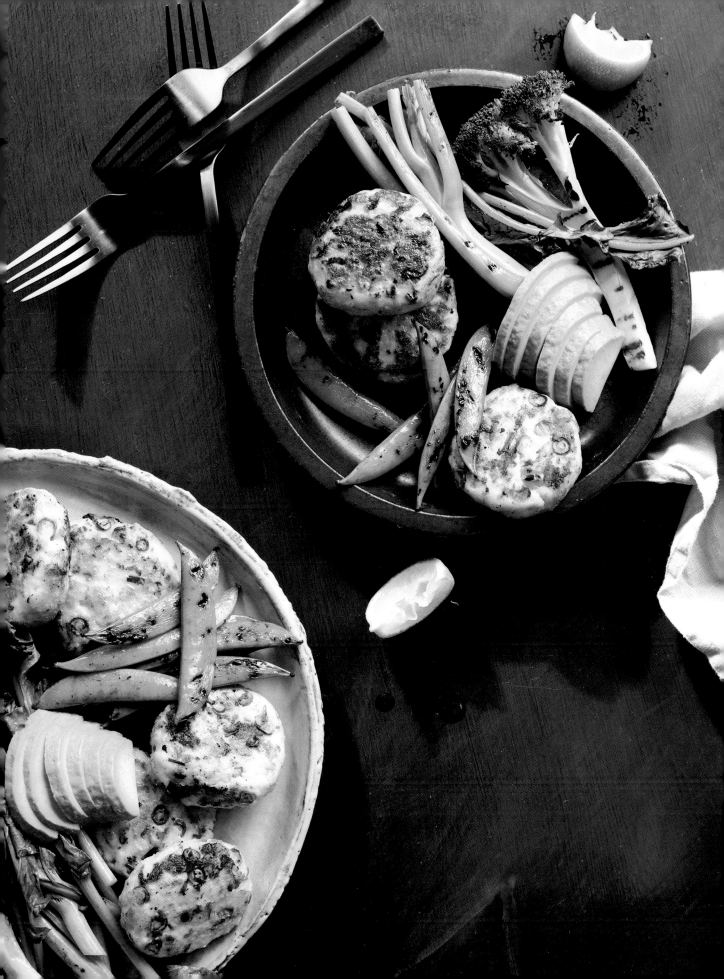

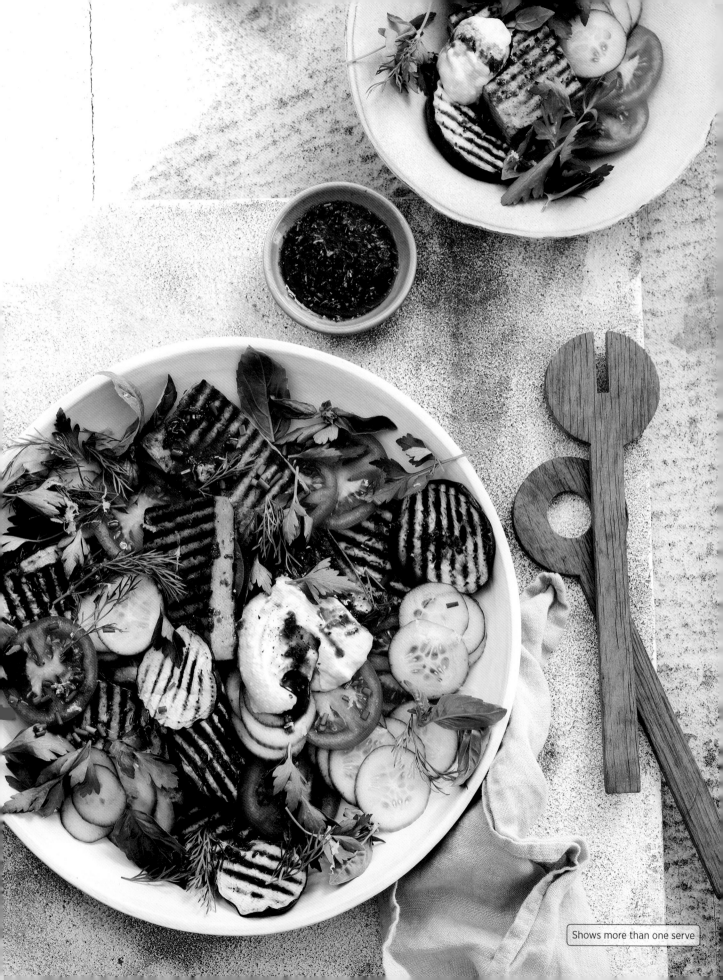

Shows more than one serve

UNITS PER SERVE

Lean meat, fish, poultry, eggs, tofu: **1.5**
Dairy and dairy alternatives: **1**
Low–moderate carb vegetables: **3**
Healthy fats: **1**

⅓ cup (80 ml) balsamic vinegar
2 cloves garlic, crushed
1 teaspoon mixed dried herbs
600 g firm tofu, cut into 8 thick
    slices (see note)
300 g eggplant, sliced into rounds

HUMMUS AND RICOTTA 'MASH'

⅓ cup (80 g) hummus
220 g ricotta
finely grated zest and juice of ½ lemon

HERB SALAD

1 cup flat-leaf parsley leaves
1 cup small basil leaves
⅓ cup dill
2 tablespoons chopped chives
300 g Lebanese cucumbers, very thinly
    sliced into rounds
300 g tomatoes, sliced into rounds
finely grated zest and juice of ½ lemon

Balsamic-glazed tofu with hummus and ricotta 'mash'

🍽 **Serves 4**   🕐 **Preparation: 30–35 minutes, plus marinating time**
🍲 **Cooking: 5 minutes**   👨‍🍳 **Difficulty: Easy**

Combine the vinegar, garlic and mixed dried herbs in a large bowl and season to taste with freshly ground black pepper. Add the tofu and toss to coat evenly. Cover and marinate in the refrigerator for at least 20 minutes.

Meanwhile, to make the hummus and ricotta 'mash', place all the ingredients in a bowl and mash until smooth and well combined. Season to taste with freshly ground black pepper. Set aside until required.

Heat a barbecue chargrill to high.

To make the herb salad, combine all the ingredients in a large bowl and season to taste with freshly ground black pepper. Set aside until required.

Add the eggplant to the tofu mixture and gently toss to combine. Season to taste with freshly ground black pepper. Chargrill the eggplant and tofu, turning occasionally, for 5 minutes or until cooked and golden.

Divide the tofu and eggplant among serving plates and drizzle with any remaining marinade. Serve with the herb salad and a good dollop of the hummus and ricotta 'mash'.

> **WEEKS 7–12 CARB EXTRAS**
>
> For an extra 7 g carbs per serve, serve with 2 (½ per person) wholemeal pita breads that have been heated through on the barbecue for 30 seconds.

Note: You can swap the tofu for 8 eggs that have been dry-fried on the barbecue flat plate for 3–4 minutes until the egg whites are set but the yolks are still soft. If you do this, use the balsamic marinade to marinate the eggplant instead.

Peri peri chargrilled chicken with mixed vegetable salad

9 G
CARB
PER
SERVE

🍴 **Serves 4**   🕐 **Preparation: 20–25 minutes, plus marinating time**
🍳 **Cooking: 15 minutes**   👩‍🍳 **Difficulty: Easy**

100 g low-fat natural
  Greek-style yoghurt
600 g lean chicken tenderloins,
  halved lengthways
2 tablespoons peri peri spice mix
300 g baby carrots, trimmed
  and scrubbed
300 g asparagus, trimmed
150 g rocket leaves, trimmed
150 g cherry tomatoes, halved
½ cup chopped curly parsley
finely grated zest and juice of 1 lemon

Combine the yoghurt, chicken and spice mix in a large bowl and season to taste with freshly ground black pepper. Cover and marinate in the refrigerator for 30 minutes.

Heat a barbecue chargrill to medium–high.

Chargrill the carrots for 3 minutes, turning occasionally, then add the asparagus and chargrill for 2 minutes. Transfer the carrot and asparagus to a large bowl. Add the rocket, tomato, parsley, lemon zest and juice and season to taste with freshly ground black pepper. Toss everything together well and set aside until required.

Chargrill the chicken, turning occasionally, for 8–10 minutes or until cooked and golden.

Serve the chicken with the salad mixture.

> **WEEKS 7–12 CARB EXTRAS**
>
> For an extra 6 g carbs per serve, serve with 2 (½ per person) wholemeal mountain bread wraps.

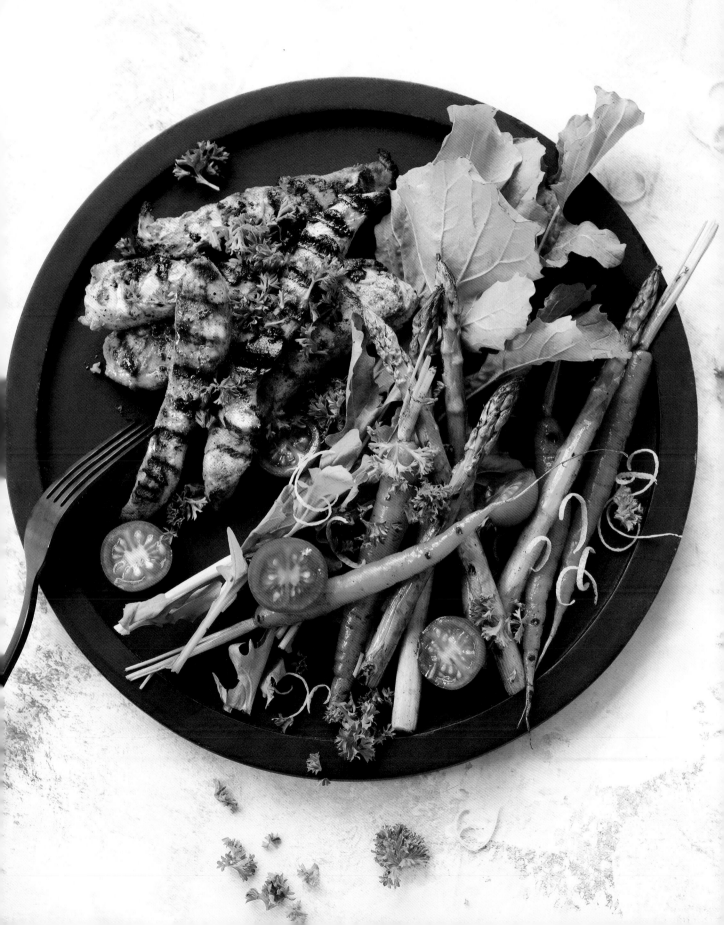

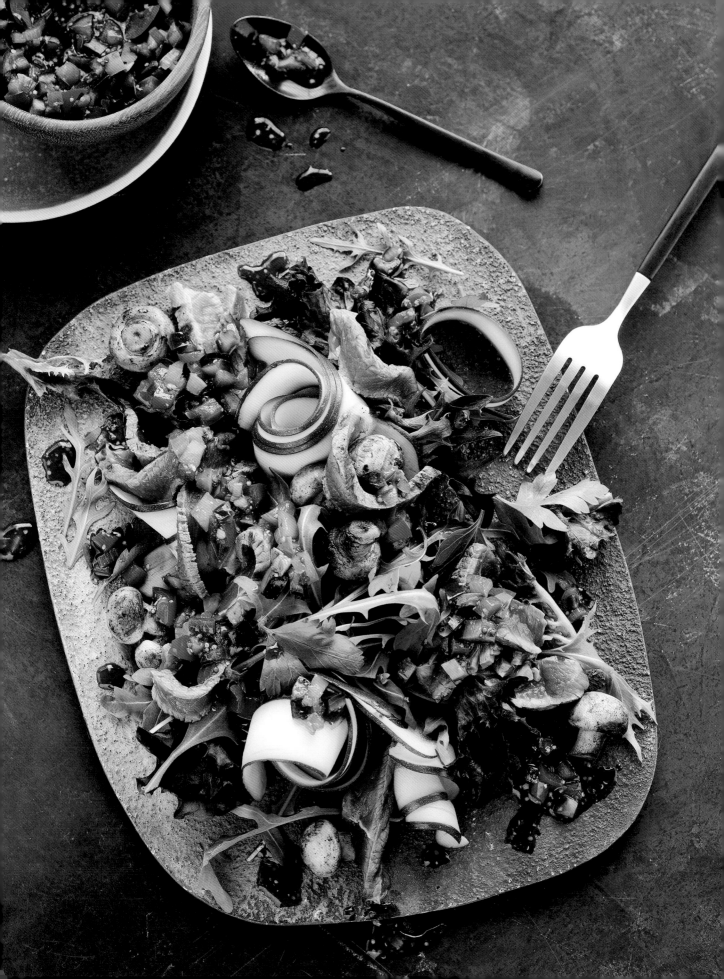

UNITS PER SERVE
Lean meat, fish, poultry, eggs, tofu: **1.5**
Low-moderate carb vegetables: **3**

Beef fillet with mushroom salad and homemade barbecue sauce

9 G
CARB
PER
SERVE

🍴 **Serves 4**   🕐 **Preparation: 20–25 minutes, plus resting time**
🍲 **Cooking: 20 minutes**   ⓢ **Difficulty: Easy**

600 g lean beef topside
300 g button mushrooms
150 g zucchini, cut with a vegetable
    peeler into long thin ribbons
75 g mixed salad leaves
50 g rocket leaves

BARBECUE SAUCE
2 cloves garlic, crushed
¼ cup (60 ml) balsamic vinegar
¼ cup (60 ml) Worcestershire sauce
1 teaspoon dried mixed herbs
2 teaspoons wholegrain mustard
150 g seeded mixed capsicums (green,
    red, yellow), finely chopped
100 g baby eggplant, finely chopped
50 g golden shallots, finely chopped

Heat a barbecue flat plate and chargrill to medium–high.

To make the barbecue sauce, mix together the garlic, vinegar, Worcestershire sauce, dried mixed herbs and mustard in a large heatproof bowl. Season to taste with freshly ground black pepper. Cook the capsicum, eggplant and shallot on the barbecue flat plate for 10 minutes or until very soft and golden. Immediately transfer the hot vegetables to the vinegar mixture in the bowl and mix well. Season to taste with freshly ground black pepper, then cover to keep warm.

Meanwhile, season the beef on all sides with freshly ground black pepper. Cook the beef on the chargrill and the mushrooms on the flat plate for 5 minutes, turning occasionally. Transfer the mushrooms to a large bowl. Cook the beef for a further 2 minutes for medium or until cooked to your liking. Transfer to a board, cover loosely with foil and rest for 5 minutes. Thinly slice the beef.

Add the zucchini, salad leaves and rocket to the mushrooms and season to taste with freshly ground black pepper. Toss well to combine.

Divide the mushroom salad among serving plates. Top with the sliced beef and barbecue sauce and serve.

WEEKS 7–12 CARB EXTRAS

For an extra 7 g carbs per serve, add 200 g (50 g per person) drained and rinsed tinned cannellini beans to the mushroom salad before serving.

Cumin lamb with pickled beetroot

1 cup flat-leaf parsley leaves
150 g cherry tomatoes, halved
150 g Lebanese cucumber, chopped
300 g small iceberg lettuce,
   cut into wedges
⅓ cup (80 g) hummus

PICKLED BEETROOT
225 g peeled beetroot, coarsely grated
1 small red onion (75 g), finely chopped
2 teaspoons wholegrain mustard
½ cup (125 ml) red wine vinegar

CUMIN LAMB
1 tablespoon cumin seeds
2 teaspoons ground coriander
1 teaspoon smoked paprika
1 tablespoon extra virgin olive oil
600 g lamb backstrap

🍴 **Serves 4** 🕐 **Preparation: 20–25 minutes, plus standing and resting time** 🍲 **Cooking: 10 minutes** 🧤 **Difficulty: Easy**

To make the pickled beetroot, mix together all the ingredients in a bowl and season to taste with freshly ground black pepper. Leave to stand at room temperature, stirring occasionally, for 30 minutes.

Heat a barbecue chargrill to high.

To make the cumin lamb, combine the spices and olive oil in a flat dish. Season to taste with freshly ground black pepper. Add the lamb and turn to coat evenly in the spiced oil on all sides. Cook on the chargrill for 3 minutes each side for medium or until cooked to your liking. Transfer to a board. Cover loosely with foil and rest for 5 minutes before slicing.

Combine the parsley, tomato and cucumber in a bowl. Divide among serving plates and add the lettuce and lamb. Serve with the hummus and pickled beetroot.

WEEKS 7–12 CARB EXTRAS

For an extra 7 g carbs per serve, serve with 2 (½ per person) wholemeal pita breads.

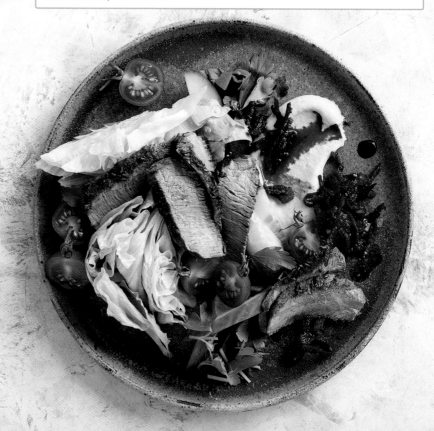

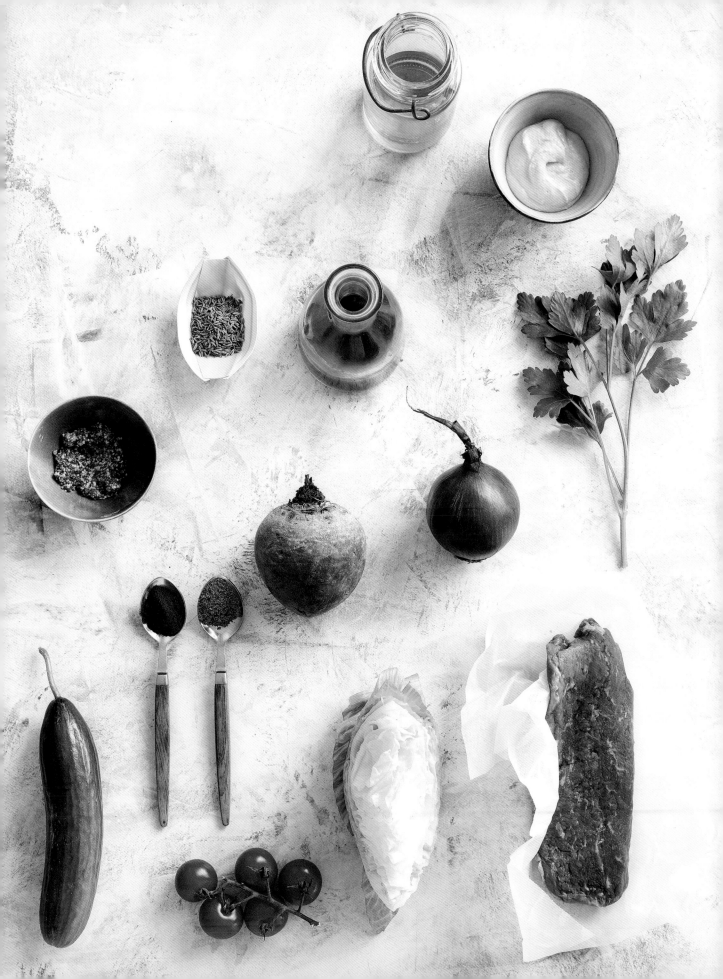

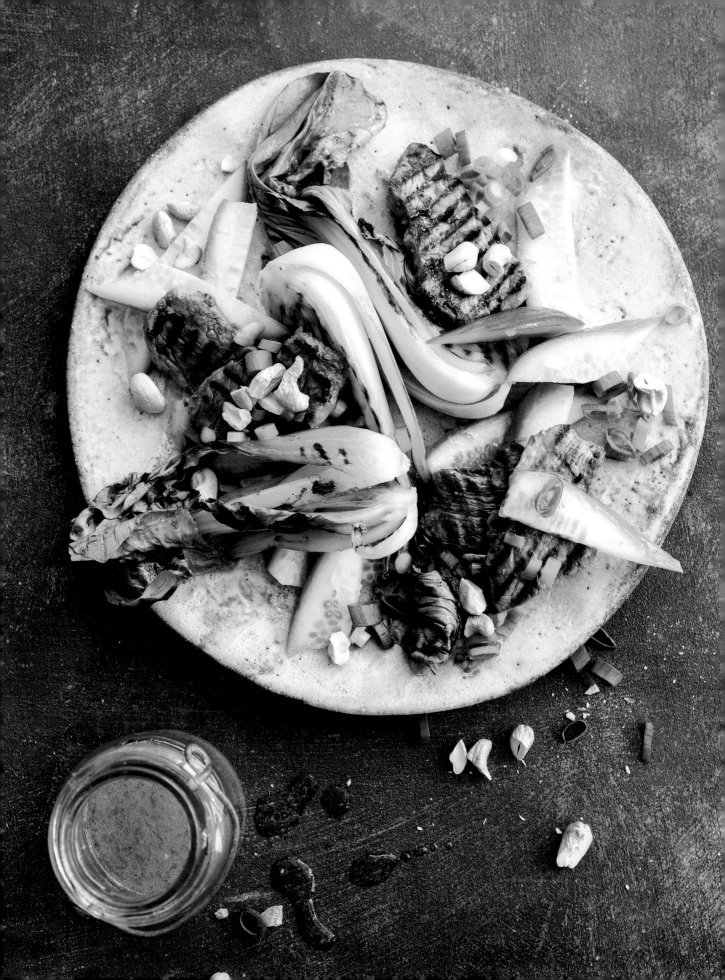

UNITS PER SERVE
Lean meat, fish, poultry, eggs, tofu: **1.5**
Low–moderate carb vegetables: **2**
Healthy fats: **2**

Hoisin pork with cashew and almond greens

11 G
CARB
PER
SERVE

🍴 **Serves 4**   🕐 **Preparation: 20–25 minutes, plus marinating time**
🍳 **Cooking: 10 minutes**   🎖 **Difficulty: Easy**

2 tablespoons hoisin sauce
¼ cup (60 ml) salt-reduced soy sauce
3 cm piece ginger, finely grated
1 clove garlic, crushed
600 g lean pork tenderloin, sinew trimmed, cut diagonally into 1 cm thick slices

CASHEW AND ALMOND GREENS

450 g baby bok choy, leaves separated
4 spring onions, thinly sliced
150 g Lebanese cucumber, quartered lengthways, sliced diagonally
finely grated zest and juice of 2 limes
1 teaspoon sesame oil
40 g raw unsalted cashews, toasted and chopped
40 g blanched almonds, toasted and chopped

Combine the hoisin, soy sauce, ginger, garlic and pork in a large glass or ceramic bowl. Season to taste with freshly ground black pepper. Cover and marinate in the refrigerator for 1 hour.

Heat a barbecue chargrill to high.

To make the cashew and almond greens, cook the bok choy, in batches, on the chargrill, turning occasionally, for 1 minute or until starting to wilt. Transfer to a bowl. Add the remaining ingredients and season to taste with freshly ground black pepper, then toss well to combine. Set aside until required.

Cook the pork on the chargrill, turning occasionally, for 6–8 minutes or until golden and cooked through.

Place the pork on serving plates and serve with the cashew greens.

WEEKS 7–12 CARB EXTRAS

For an extra 8 g carbs per serve, serve with 200 g (50 g per person) cooked quinoa.

Note: You can marinate the pork for up to 2 days before you cook it, if desired. Just give the mixture a stir every day.

UNITS PER SERVE
Lean meat, fish, poultry, eggs, tofu: **1.5**
Low-moderate carb vegetables: **4**
Healthy fats: **3.5**

Fish finger skewers with warm vegetable salad

9 G
CARB
PER
SERVE

🍽 **Serves 4**   🕐 **Preparation: 30–35 minutes**
🍳 **Cooking: 10 minutes**   👨‍🍳 **Difficulty: Easy**

finely grated zest and juice of 1 lemon
2 teaspoons Dijon mustard
2 tablespoons finely chopped chives
¼ cup dill
600 g thick white fish fillets, skin
    removed, pin-boned and cut into
    2 cm wide strips
1 lemon, extra, cut into wedges

VEGETABLE SALAD

2 tablespoons white wine vinegar
2 tablespoons extra virgin olive oil
pinch saffron threads, optional
150 g mixed baby tomatoes, halved
300 g small yellow squash,
    halved horizontally
300 g baby fennel, trimmed, thickly
    sliced lengthways
300 g broccolini, trimmed, halved
    lengthways
150 g rocket leaves
60 g whole natural almonds, toasted
    and chopped

Heat a barbecue chargrill to medium–high.

To make the vegetable salad, combine the vinegar, olive oil, saffron (if using) and tomato in a bowl. Use a potato masher to squash the tomato slightly and season to taste with freshly ground black pepper. Set aside. Chargrill the squash, fennel and broccolini, turning occasionally, for 5 minutes or until just tender and golden. Immediately transfer to a heatproof bowl and toss well to combine. Add the rocket and almonds and toss again.

Place the lemon zest and juice, mustard, chives, dill and fish in a large bowl and gently toss to coat on all sides. Season to taste with freshly ground black pepper. Thread the fish strips evenly onto 12 metal skewers.

Chargrill the fish skewers, turning occasionally, for 5 minutes or until just cooked and golden.

Divide the vegetable salad among four plates and top with the fish skewers. Serve with the tomato mixture and extra lemon wedges.

> **WEEKS 7–12 CARB EXTRAS**
>
> For an extra 9 g carbs per serve, add 160 g (40 g per person) cooked puy lentils to the vegetable salad mixture.

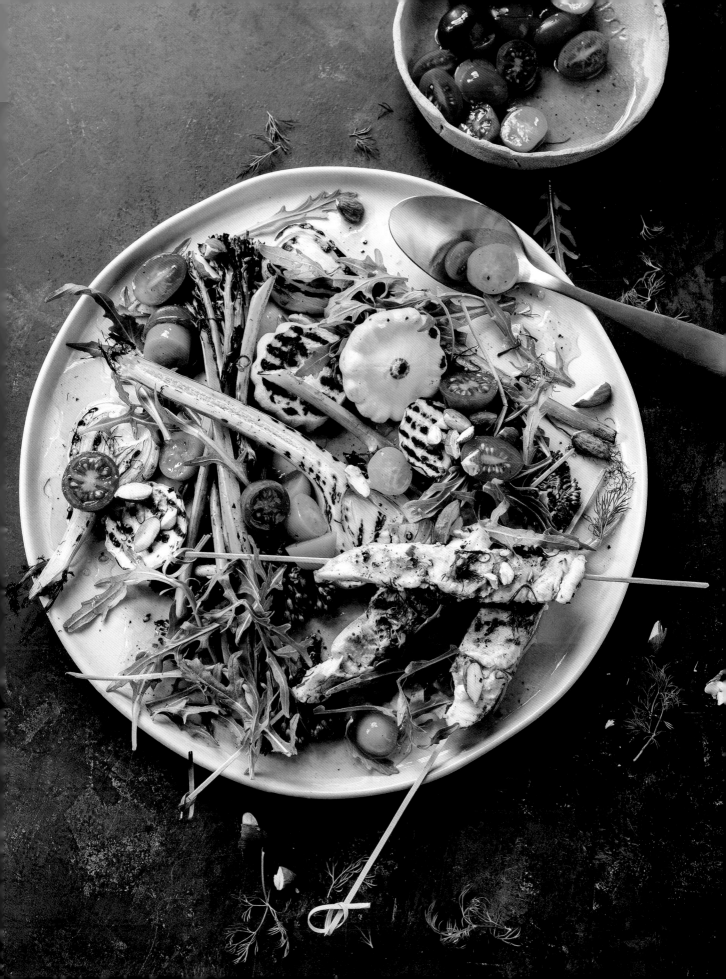

WEEKEND MEALS

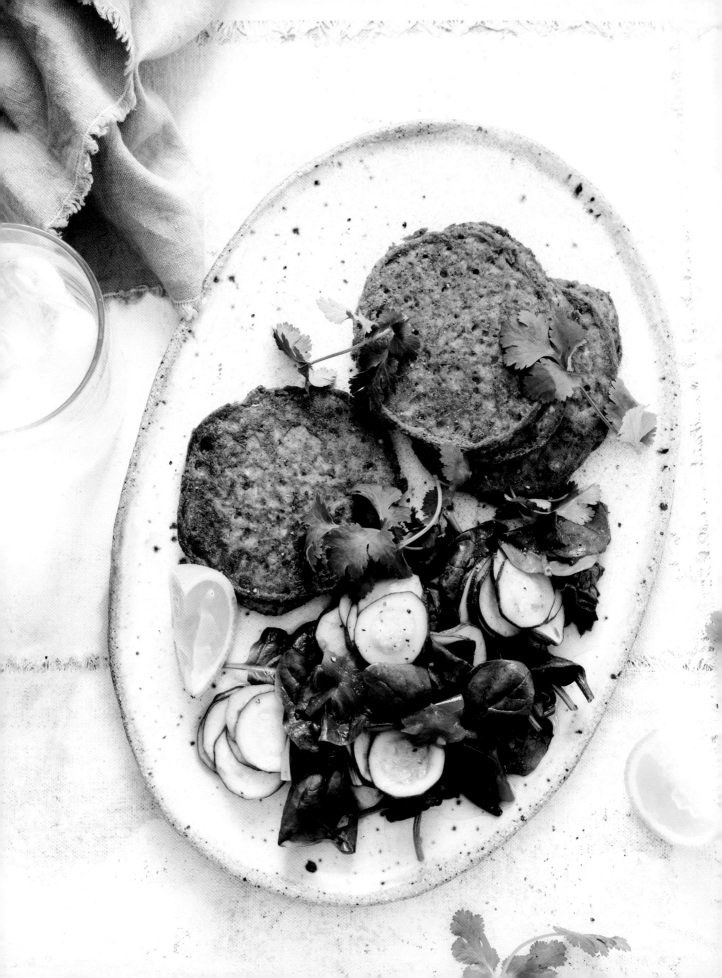

Tofu falafel fritters with braised greens

10 G CARB PER SERVE

🍴 Serves 4   🕐 Preparation: 25–30 minutes
🍲 Cooking: 20 minutes   👨‍🍳 Difficulty: Medium

160 g drained and rinsed
   tinned chickpeas
200 g firm tofu, finely chopped
1 cup flat-leaf parsley leaves
2 cloves garlic, roughly chopped
1 tablespoon tahini
finely grated zest of 1 lemon
2 teaspoons sweet paprika
3 teaspoons garam masala
4 eggs
2 tablespoons rice bran oil

BRAISED GREENS
1 tablespoon olive oil
200 g tomatoes, chopped
300 g zucchini, very thinly sliced
   into rounds
½ cup (125 ml) salt-reduced
   vegetable stock
100 g baby spinach leaves
½ cup coriander leaves
juice of 1 lemon

Process the chickpeas, tofu, parsley, garlic, tahini, lemon zest, paprika and garam masala in a food processor until smooth and well combined. Add the eggs and process until well combined. Season to taste with freshly ground black pepper.

Heat the rice bran oil in a large frying pan over medium–high heat. Working in batches, add 2 tablespoon measures of the mixture and cook for 3–4 minutes each side or until golden and cooked through. Transfer to a plate and cover to keep warm. You will have enough mixture to make 12 fritters.

Meanwhile, to make the braised greens, heat the olive oil in a large saucepan over medium heat. Add the tomato and zucchini and cook, stirring occasionally, for 3 minutes or until starting to soften. Add the stock and cook, stirring occasionally, for 10 minutes or until the vegetables are very tender and the stock has reduced by half. Add the spinach in batches, stirring until wilted before adding the next batch. Remove the pan from the heat and season to taste with freshly ground black pepper. Stir in the coriander and lemon juice.

Serve the fritters with the braised greens.

WEEKS 7–12 CARB EXTRAS

For an extra 9 g carbs per serve, add 200 g (50 g per person) peeled and chopped sweet potato to the braised greens when you add the tomato and zucchini.

Zucchini and ricotta pie with avocado and pecan salad

7 G
CARB
PER
SERVE

🍴 **Serves 4**　🕐 **Preparation: 30–35 minutes**
🌀 **Cooking: 40 minutes**　👨‍🍳 **Difficulty: Medium**

UNITS PER SERVE
Lean meat, fish, poultry, eggs, tofu: **1**
Dairy and dairy alternatives: **1**
Low–moderate carb vegetables: **3**
Healthy fats: **4**

200 g silken tofu
4 eggs
220 g ricotta
2 tablespoons thyme leaves
2 tablespoons chopped chives
600 g yellow and green zucchini,
　cut with a vegetable peeler into
　long thin ribbons
olive oil spray, for cooking
240 g avocado, sliced
½ cup flat-leaf parsley leaves
finely grated zest and juice of 1 lemon
40 g pecans, toasted and
　roughly chopped

Preheat the oven to 200°C (180°C fan-forced). Line the base and sides of a 28 cm x 18 cm baking tin with baking paper.

Process the tofu, eggs, ricotta, thyme and chives in a food processor until well combined. Season to taste with freshly ground black pepper. Pour the mixture into the prepared tin and level the surface.

Tightly roll up each piece of zucchini and press it firmly into the ricotta mixture. Be sure to place the zucchini rolls close together in the tin. Spray lightly with olive oil and bake for 40 minutes or until set and golden. Rest in the tin for 5 minutes before removing.

Carefully toss the avocado, parsley, lemon zest and juice and chopped pecans in a bowl. Season to taste with freshly ground black pepper. Slice the zucchini pie and serve with the salad.

WEEKS 7–12 CARB EXTRAS

For an extra 9 g carbs per serve, add 160 g (40 g per person) drained and rinsed tinned brown lentils to the salad.

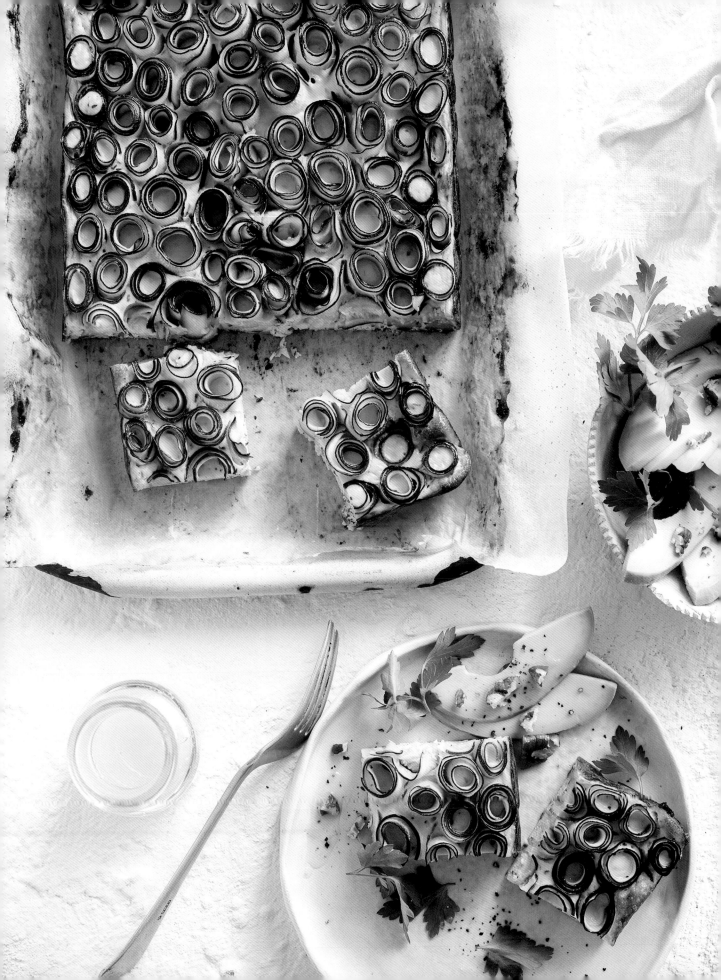

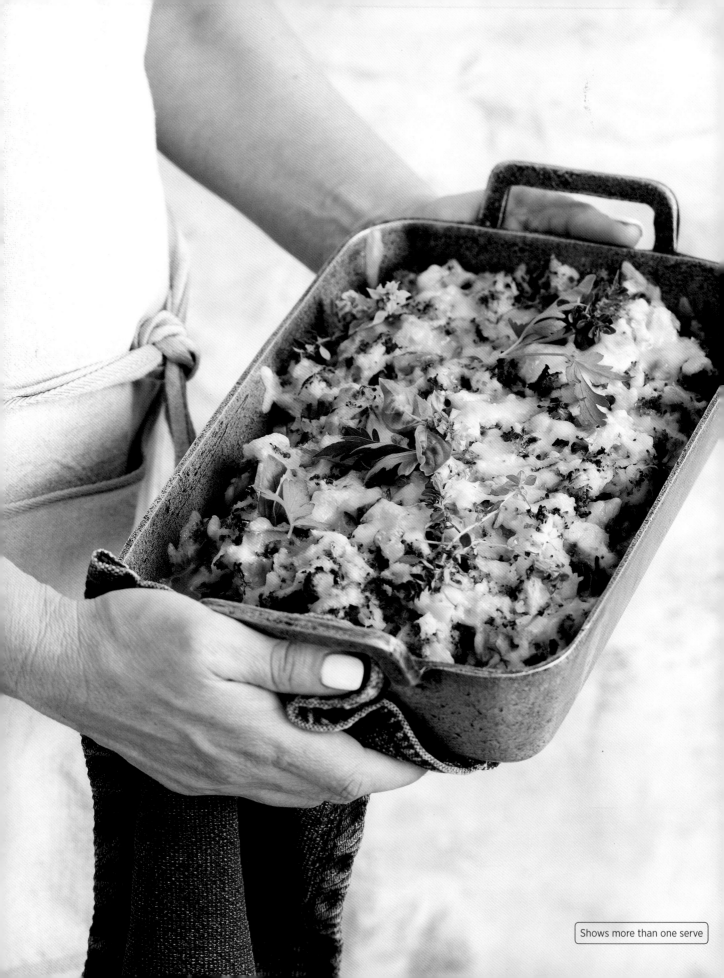

Shows more than one serve

Chicken and lentil cottage pie

13 G
CARB
PER
SERVE

🍴 Serves 4   🕐 Preparation: 25–30 minutes
🍲 Cooking: 20 minutes   🍳 Difficulty: Medium

1 tablespoon olive oil
400 g lean chicken breast
    fillets, chopped
2 cloves garlic, crushed
320 g drained and rinsed tinned lentils
2 tablespoons lemon thyme leaves,
    plus extra to serve
1 tablespoon finely chopped rosemary
2 cups (500 ml) salt-reduced
    chicken stock
1 cup small basil leaves, plus extra
    to serve
½ cup chopped flat-leaf parsley,
    plus extra leaves to serve
80 g cheddar, finely grated

MASH
300 g broccoli florets, chopped
300 g peeled celeriac, chopped
2 tablespoons olive oil margarine
2 tablespoons chopped chives

Heat the olive oil in a large saucepan over high heat. Add the chicken and garlic and cook, stirring occasionally, for 3 minutes or until light golden. Add the lentils, thyme, rosemary and stock and cook, stirring occasionally, for 10 minutes or until cooked through and the sauce has reduced by half. Remove the pan from the heat. Stir in the basil and parsley and season to taste with freshly ground black pepper.

Meanwhile, to make the mash, steam the broccoli and celeriac together for 10 minutes or until tender. Transfer to a bowl. Add the margarine and mash until smooth. Stir in the chives and season to taste with freshly ground black pepper.

Preheat the oven grill to high. Spoon the chicken mixture into a 5 cm deep, 20 cm x 12 cm flameproof baking dish. Top with the mash and sprinkle evenly with the cheese. Cook under the grill for 4–5 minutes or until bubbling and golden. Rest for 5 minutes, then serve topped with the extra lemon thyme, basil and parsley leaves.

WEEKS 7–12 CARB EXTRAS

For an extra 6 g carbs per serve, add 200 g (50 g per person) pumpkin to the steamer with the broccoli and celeriac when making the mash.

Pistachio-crumbed barramundi with baked vegetables

12 G CARB PER SERVE

🍽 **Serves 4** 🕐 **Preparation: 20–25 minutes**
🍲 **Cooking: 25 minutes** ⓦ **Difficulty: Medium**

150 g baby fennel, thinly sliced
    lengthways
1 red onion (150 g), cut into thin wedges
300 g small yellow squash, quartered
250 g cherry tomatoes, halved
2 tablespoons olive oil
1 teaspoon ground turmeric
1 teaspoon garlic powder
4 x 150 g barramundi fillets, skin
    removed and pin-boned
50 g baby rocket leaves

PISTACHIO CRUMB

80 g unsalted shelled pistachios,
    finely chopped
1 clove garlic, crushed
finely grated zest and juice of 1 lemon
2 tablespoons small oregano leaves
1 tablespoon thyme leaves

Preheat the oven to 200°C (180°C fan-forced).

Combine the fennel, onion, squash, tomato, olive oil, turmeric, garlic powder and ⅓ cup (80 ml) water in a large heavy-based baking dish. Season to taste with freshly ground black pepper. Rest the barramundi on top and season with more black pepper.

To make the pistachio crumb, combine all the ingredients in a small bowl and season to taste with freshly ground black pepper. Press the mixture evenly over the barramundi.

Bake for 25 minutes or until cooked through and golden. Carefully transfer the barramundi to serving plates. Add the rocket to the vegetable mixture in the dish and toss well to combine. Serve with the barramundi.

> **WEEKS 7–12 CARB EXTRAS**
>
> For an extra 9 g carbs per serve, add 200 g (50 g per person) peeled and sliced sweet potato to the vegetables before baking.

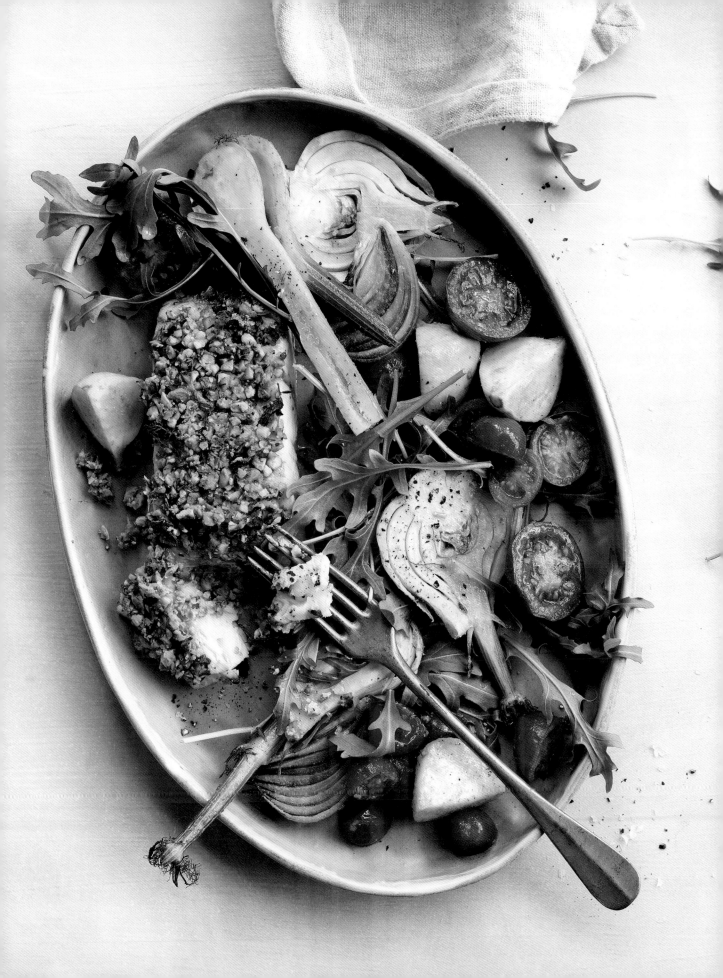

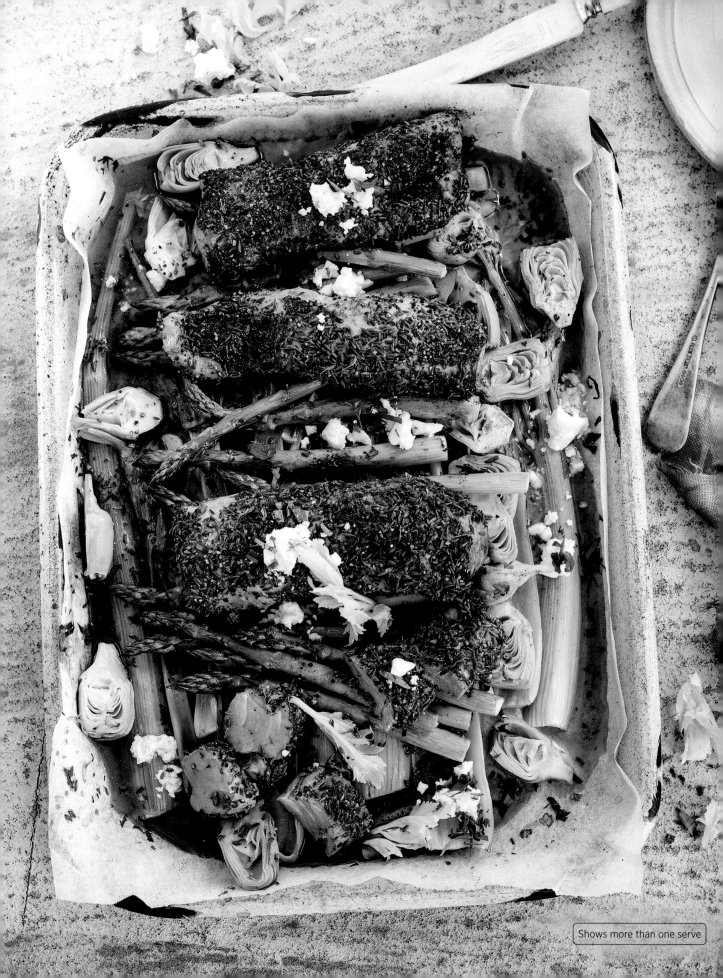

Shows more than one serve

Roast pork with celery, artichokes and feta

8 G CARB PER SERVE

UNITS PER SERVE

Lean meat, fish, poultry, eggs, tofu: **1.5**
Dairy and dairy alternatives: **1**
Low–moderate carb vegetables: **3**
Healthy fats: **1**

🍽 **Serves 4**   🕐 **Preparation: 25–30 minutes**
🍲 **Cooking: 30 minutes**   ⚙ **Difficulty: Medium**

300 g celery heart, stalks separated and ends trimmed, large green leaves discarded, inner yellow leaves reserved

1 cup flat-leaf parsley leaves, plus 2 tablespoons finely chopped flat-leaf parsley, extra

2 cloves garlic, sliced

1 cup (250 ml) salt-reduced chicken stock

300 g drained artichoke hearts in brine, halved lengthways

300 g asparagus, trimmed

1 tablespoon olive oil

600 g lean pork tenderloin, sinew removed, cut crossways into 4 equal portions

2 tablespoons freshly ground black pepper

2 tablespoons cumin seeds

2 teaspoons sweet paprika

80 g Greek feta, coarsely crumbled

Preheat the oven to 220°C (200°C fan-forced).

Combine the celery stalks, parsley leaves, garlic and stock in a large heavy-based baking dish. Cover tightly with foil and roast for 15 minutes. Carefully remove from the oven and add the artichoke and asparagus.

Rub the olive oil all over the pork portions. Sprinkle the pepper, cumin and paprika over a large board and toss to combine. Roll the pork portions over the mixture to evenly coat on all sides. Rest the pork on top of the vegetables in the dish and roast, uncovered, for 15 minutes or until cooked and golden. Remove from the oven, cover loosely with foil and rest for 5 minutes.

Combine the feta, extra parsley and reserved yellow celery leaves in a small bowl and season to taste with freshly ground black pepper. Sprinkle over the pork and vegetable mixture and serve.

WEEKS 7–12 CARB EXTRAS

For an extra 8 g carbs per serve, add 200 g (50 g per person) cooked quinoa to the roasted vegetables in the dish, then toss to combine and heat through before serving.

Roast chicken with whipped ricotta

UNITS PER SERVE
Lean meat, fish, poultry, eggs, tofu: **1.5**
Dairy and dairy alternatives: **1**
Low–moderate carb vegetables: **3**
Healthy fats: **2**

🍴 **Serves 4**　🕐 **Preparation: 25–30 minutes**
🍲 **Cooking: 30 minutes**　🍳 **Difficulty: Medium**

150 g peeled parsnip, thinly
　sliced lengthways
150 g baby carrots, trimmed
　and scrubbed
300 g peeled celeriac or zucchini
　(unpeeled), cut into batons
300 g broccolini, trimmed and
　halved lengthways
2 lemons, skin and white pith removed,
　sliced into rounds (see note)
4 x 150 g lean chicken breast fillets
3 teaspoons celery seeds
2 tablespoons lemon thyme leaves
40 g slivered almonds
1 tablespoon extra virgin olive oil

WHIPPED RICOTTA
200 g ricotta
¼ cup (20 g) finely grated parmesan
3 teaspoons finely grated lemon zest
1 tablespoon drained capers in brine,
　rinsed and chopped
2 tablespoons chopped chives

Preheat the oven to 220°C (200°C fan-forced).

Combine the parsnip, carrots, celeriac, broccolini, lemon and ½ cup (125 ml) water in a large heavy-based baking dish and rest the chicken on top. Sprinkle with the celery seeds, lemon thyme and almonds, drizzle over the olive oil and season to taste with freshly ground black pepper. Roast for 30 minutes or until cooked through and golden. Remove and cover loosely with foil, then rest for 5 minutes.

Meanwhile, to make the whipped ricotta, whip the ricotta, parmesan, lemon zest and 1 tablespoon water together with hand-held beaters for 2 minutes or until completely smooth and aerated. Stir through the capers and chives and season to taste with freshly ground black pepper.

Serve the roast chicken and vegetables with the whipped ricotta.

WEEKS 7–12 CARB EXTRAS

For an extra 8 g carbs per serve, serve with 200 g (50 g per person) cooked quinoa.

Note: Be sure to finely grate the lemon zest from the lemons required for roasting before peeling and discarding their skins. You will use the grated zest in the whipped ricotta.

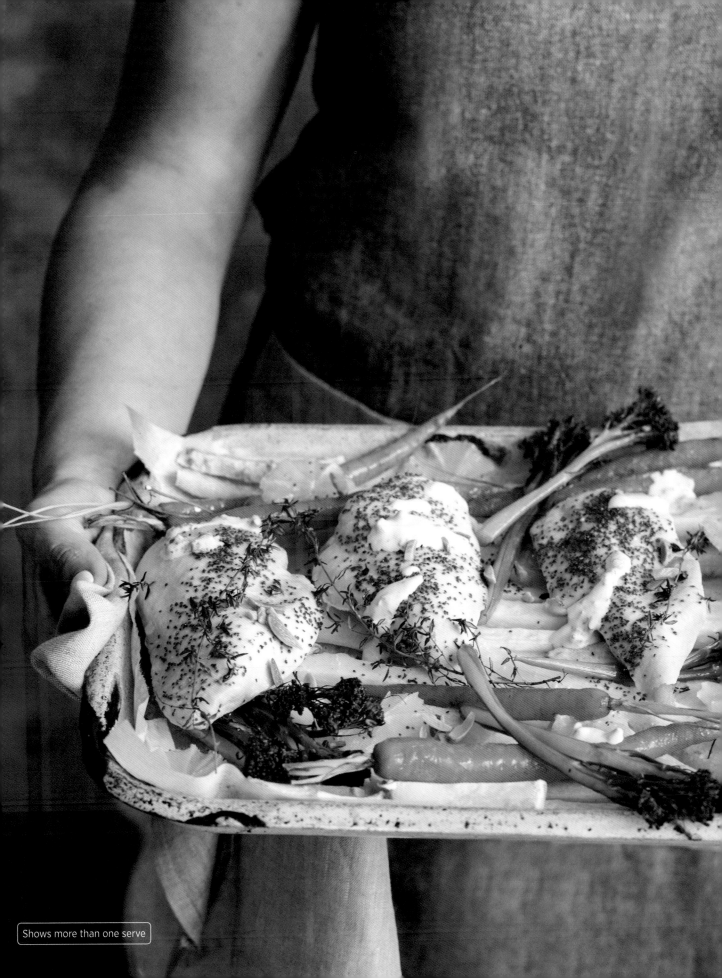

Shows more than one serve

Beef and vegetable lasagne

UNITS PER SERVE

Lean meat, fish, poultry, eggs, tofu: **1.5**
Dairy and dairy alternatives: **1**
Low–moderate carb vegetables: **4**

🍴 **Serves 4** 🕐 **Preparation: 35–40 minutes**
🍲 **Cooking: 1 hour** 🍳 **Difficulty: Medium**

300 g eggplant, thinly sliced
   into rounds
400 g zucchini, cut with a vegetable
   peeler into long thin ribbons
600 g lean beef eye fillet, chopped
2 cloves garlic, roughly chopped
2 teaspoons dried thyme
1 teaspoon dried rosemary
1 cup (250 ml) tomato passata
1 cup (250 ml) salt-reduced beef stock
100 g mozzarella, finely grated

DRESSED GREENS

2 tablespoons balsamic vinegar
1 teaspoon Dijon mustard
50 g mixed salad leaves
150 g Lebanese cucumber,
   thinly sliced into rounds
½ cup small flat-leaf parsley leaves

Preheat the oven to 200°C (180°C fan-forced).

Heat a chargrill pan over high heat. Add the eggplant and zucchini in batches and cook, turning once, for 2 minutes each or until just softened and golden. Transfer to a plate.

Process the beef, garlic, thyme and rosemary in a food processor until finely minced.

Heat a large non-stick frying pan over high heat. Add the beef mixture and cook for 10 minutes until golden, breaking up any large lumps with the back of a spoon. Add the passata and stock and cook, stirring occasionally, for 15 minutes or until the sauce has reduced by half. Season to taste with freshly ground black pepper.

Layer the beef mixture, eggplant and zucchini in a 6 cm deep, 28 cm x 18 cm baking dish. Sprinkle the mozzarella over the top and bake for 25 minutes or until bubbling and golden. Remove and rest for 5 minutes.

Meanwhile, to make the dressed greens, whisk together the vinegar and mustard in a large bowl. Add the remaining ingredients and season to taste with freshly ground black pepper. Toss well to combine.

Serve the lasagne with the dressed greens.

> **WEEKS 7–12 CARB EXTRAS**
>
> For an extra 9 g carbs per serve, add 200 g (50 g per person) peeled and coarsely grated sweet potato while cooking the beef and passata mixture.

Ratatouille with egg and macadamia haloumi crust

12 G CARB PER SERVE

UNITS PER SERVE
Lean meat, fish, poultry, eggs, tofu: **1.5**
Dairy and dairy alternatives: **1**
Low–moderate carb vegetables: **5**
Healthy fats: **2**

🍴 Serves 4   🕐 Preparation: 25–30 minutes
🍳 Cooking: 45 minutes   👐 Difficulty: Medium

1 x 300 g jar mild salsa
150 g small cauliflower florets
150 g eggplant, chopped
300 g cap mushrooms
300 g zucchini, thickly sliced
1 cup (250 ml) salt-reduced
    vegetable stock
2 teaspoons dried mixed herbs
12 eggs
80 g haloumi, finely chopped
80 g macadamias, finely chopped
1 cup small basil leaves
2 tablespoons small oregano leaves

Preheat the oven to 200°C (180°C fan-forced).

Combine the salsa, cauliflower, eggplant, mushrooms, zucchini, stock and dried mixed herbs in a heavy-based baking dish. Season to taste with freshly ground black pepper, then cover and bake for 30 minutes or until the vegetables are tender.

Meanwhile, cook the eggs in a large saucepan of boiling water for 8 minutes. Drain and cool slightly, then peel and halve lengthways. Set aside until required.

Preheat the oven to 220°C (200°C fan-forced).

Rest the eggs in the vegetable mixture and sprinkle with the combined haloumi, macadamias, basil and oregano. Season to taste with freshly ground black pepper. Bake, uncovered, for 12 minutes or until golden. Serve warm.

WEEKS 7-12 CARB EXTRAS

For an extra 9 g carbs per serve, add 160 g (40 g per person) drained and rinsed tinned brown lentils to the vegetable mixture just before you add the egg.

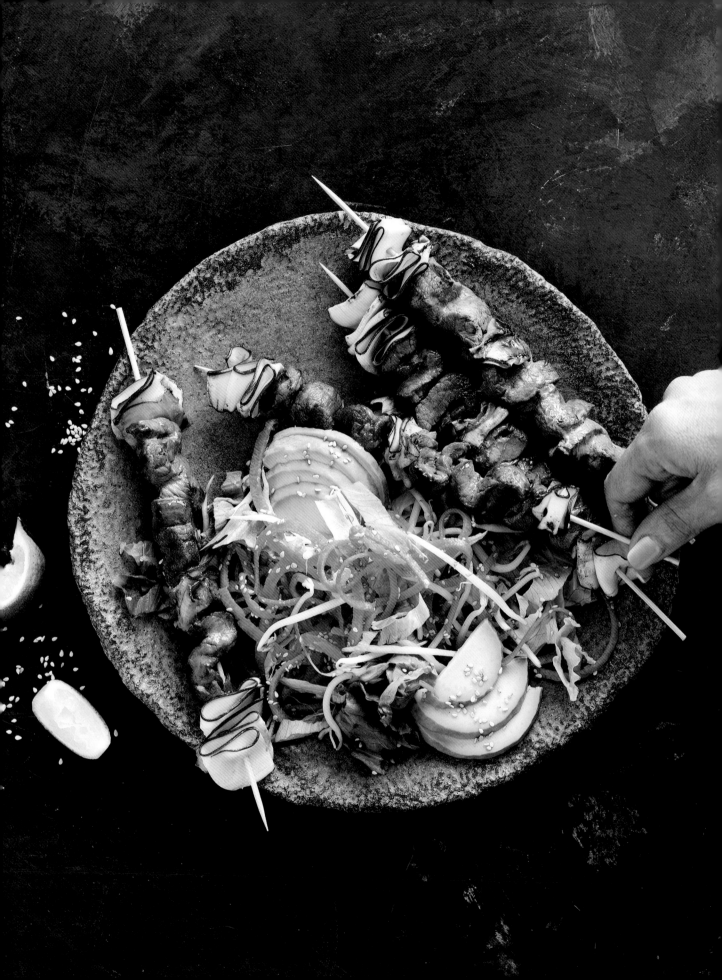

Teriyaki beef skewers with sesame carrot noodles

8 G CARB PER SERVE

🍴 **Serves 4** 🕐 **Preparation: 30–35 minutes, plus marinating time**
♨ **Cooking: 10 minutes** 👨‍🍳 **Difficulty: Medium**

1 tablespoon oyster sauce
¼ cup (60 ml) salt-reduced soy sauce
2 cloves garlic, crushed
600 g lean beef fillet, cut into
   long strips
300 g zucchini, cut with a vegetable
   peeler into long thin ribbons
160 g avocado, sliced
lime wedges, to serve

SESAME CARROT NOODLES

300 g carrot, spiralised into long
   thin noodles
2 tablespoons white wine vinegar
1 teaspoon sesame oil
50 g bean sprouts, trimmed
¼ cup (35 g) toasted sesame seeds
250 g iceberg lettuce, shredded

Combine the oyster sauce, soy sauce, garlic and beef in a glass or ceramic bowl. Season to taste with freshly ground black pepper. Cover and marinate in the refrigerator for at least 2 hours, or overnight if time permits.

Heat a large chargrill pan over medium heat. Thread the beef and zucchini ribbons onto 12 metal skewers. Cook on the chargrill, turning occasionally, for 8 minutes or until just tender and golden.

Meanwhile, to make the sesame carrot noodles, combine all the ingredients in a bowl. Season to taste with freshly ground black pepper, then set aside until required.

Divide the avocado among serving plates. Add the beef skewers and sesame carrot noodles and serve with lime wedges.

WEEKS 7–12 CARB EXTRAS

For an extra 8 g carbs per serve, serve with 200 g (50 g per person) cooked quinoa.

Lamb and vegetable massaman curry

UNITS PER SERVE
Lean meat, fish, poultry, eggs, tofu: **1.5**
Low–moderate carb vegetables: **3**
Healthy fats: **4**

🍴 **Serves 4**   🕐 **Preparation: 30–35 minutes**
🍲 **Cooking: 15 minutes**   👨‍🍳 **Difficulty: Medium**

1 tablespoon rice bran oil
600 g lamb backstrap, cut into
    2 cm pieces
300 g carrots, halved lengthways
    and sliced diagonally
300 g zucchini, halved lengthways
    and sliced diagonally
300 g tomatoes, chopped
3 cups (750 ml) salt-reduced beef stock
½ cup coriander leaves
½ cup small Thai basil leaves (see note)

CURRY PASTE
120 g blanched almonds
2 cloves garlic, roughly chopped
3 cm piece ginger, peeled
1 fresh long red chilli, chopped
3 teaspoons ground cardamom
1 teaspoon ground cinnamon
2 teaspoons ground cumin

To make the curry paste, place all the ingredients in a food processor and process until a paste forms, adding 1–2 tablespoons water if needed. Set aside until required.

Heat half the rice bran oil in a large wok over high heat. Add the lamb in three batches and stir-fry for 1 minute each. Transfer to a large bowl.

Heat the remaining oil in the same wok over high heat, add the curry paste and stir-fry for 4 minutes or until fragrant and deep golden. Add the carrot, zucchini and tomato and stir-fry for 3 minutes or until the tomato starts to collapse.

Add the stock and cook, stirring occasionally, for 3 minutes or until reduced by one-third. Return the lamb and any juices to the wok and cook, tossing, for 30 seconds.

Divide the lamb among bowls and serve topped with the coriander and Thai basil.

WEEKS 7–12 CARB EXTRAS

For an extra 8 g carbs per serve, serve with 480 g (120 g per person) steamed baby green peas.

Note: Swap the Thai basil for regular basil leaves, if desired.

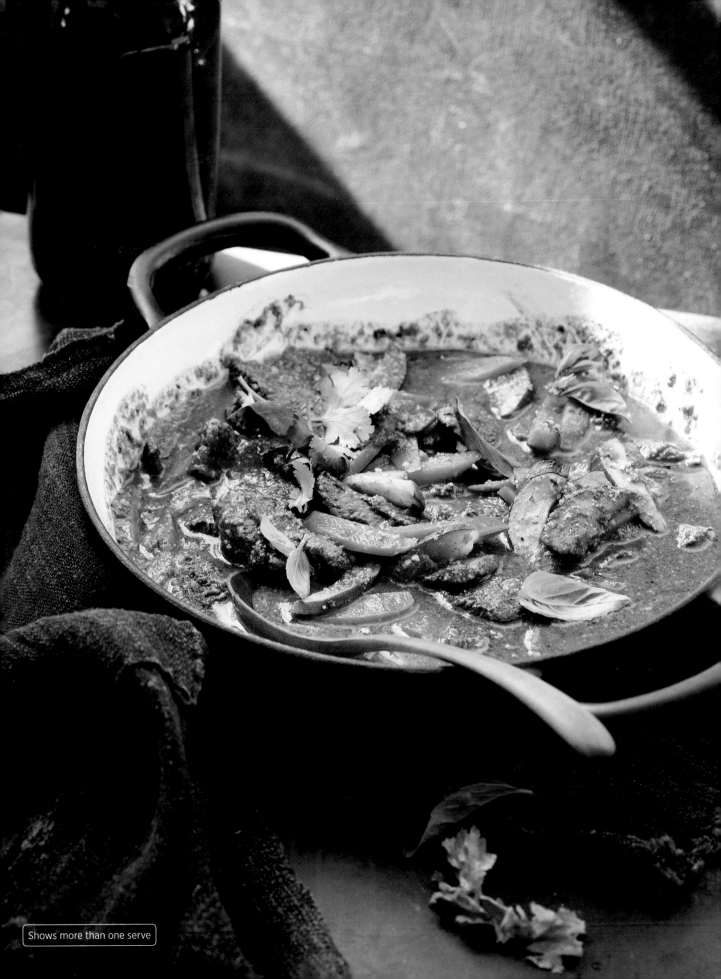

Shows more than one serve

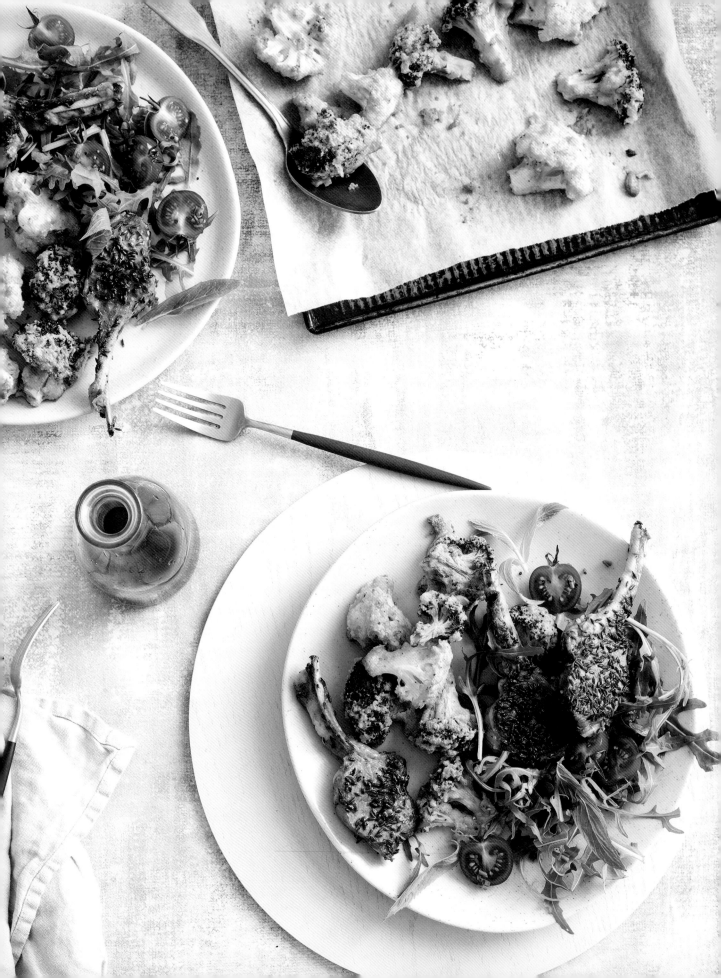

Lamb with popcorn broccoli and cauliflower

6 G
CARB
PER
SERVE

UNITS PER SERVE

Lean meat, fish, poultry, eggs, tofu: **1.5**

Low–moderate carb vegetables: **3**

Healthy fats: **2**

🍴 **Serves 4** 🕐 **Preparation: 20–25 minutes**
🍳 **Cooking: 20 minutes** 👨‍🍳 **Difficulty: Medium**

1 tablespoon cumin seeds

500 g French-trimmed lamb cutlets

50 g baby rocket leaves

250 g cherry tomatoes, halved

2 tablespoons chopped chives

¼ cup chopped mint

2 tablespoons red wine vinegar

**POPCORN BROCCOLI
AND CAULIFLOWER**

2 eggs

80 g ground almonds

3 teaspoons all-purpose seasoning

300 g small broccoli florets

300 g small cauliflower florets

To make the popcorn broccoli and cauliflower, preheat the oven to 220°C (200°C fan-forced) and line a baking tray with baking paper. Whisk the eggs in a large bowl and season to taste with freshly ground black pepper. Add the remaining ingredients and toss until well combined and coated. Spread evenly over the prepared tray and roast, turning once, for 15–20 minutes or until crisp and golden.

Meanwhile, heat a chargrill pan over high heat. Sprinkle the cumin seeds over both sides of the lamb cutlets and season to taste with freshly ground black pepper. Chargrill the cutlets for 2 minutes each side for medium or until cooked to your liking. Transfer to a plate, cover loosely with foil and rest for 5 minutes.

Combine the rocket, tomato, chives, mint and vinegar in a bowl and season to taste with freshly ground black pepper. Divide the salad and popcorn broccoli and cauliflower among serving plates. Add the lamb, drizzle with any juices, and serve.

> **WEEKS 7–12 CARB EXTRAS**
>
> For an extra 8 g carbs per serve, add 200 g (50 g per person) cooked quinoa to the salad before serving.

Thai chicken and supergreens curry

8 G
CARB
PER
SERVE

🍽 **Serves 4** 🕐 **Preparation: 25–30 minutes**
🍲 **Cooking: 10 minutes** 👨‍🍳 **Difficulty: Medium**

1 tablespoon rice bran oil
600 g lean chicken breast fillets,
    thinly sliced
100 g green beans, trimmed
200 g broccolini, trimmed and cut
    into 5 cm lengths
150 g sugar snap peas, trimmed
    and halved
150 g Chinese broccoli, trimmed
150 g kale leaves, white stalk
    removed, torn
2 cups (500 ml) salt-reduced
    chicken stock
75 g bean sprouts, trimmed
lime wedges, to serve

CURRY PASTE

80 g macadamias
2 cloves garlic, roughly chopped
4 cm piece ginger, peeled
2 stalks lemongrass,
    white part only, chopped
2 kaffir lime leaves, shredded
2 fresh long green chillies, chopped
4 spring onions, cut into 3 cm lengths
1 cup coriander leaves
25 g baby spinach leaves

To make the curry paste, place all the ingredients and ⅓ cup (80 ml) water in a food processor and process until a paste forms. Set aside until required.

Heat the rice bran oil in a large wok over high heat, add the chicken and stir-fry for 3 minutes. Add the curry paste and stir-fry for 1 minute or until fragrant. Add the beans and broccolini and cook, tossing, for 3 minutes or until almost tender. Add the sugar snap peas, Chinese broccoli, kale and stock and stir-fry for 3 minutes or until the leaves have wilted and the sauce has reduced by one-third. Season to taste with freshly ground black pepper.

Serve the curry topped with the bean sprouts, with lime wedges on the side.

WEEKS 7–12 CARB EXTRAS

For an extra 8 g carbs per serve, serve with 200 g (50 g per person) cooked quinoa.

Note: Make it a vegetarian curry by swapping the chicken for the same quantity of diced firm tofu and replacing the chicken stock with vegetable stock.

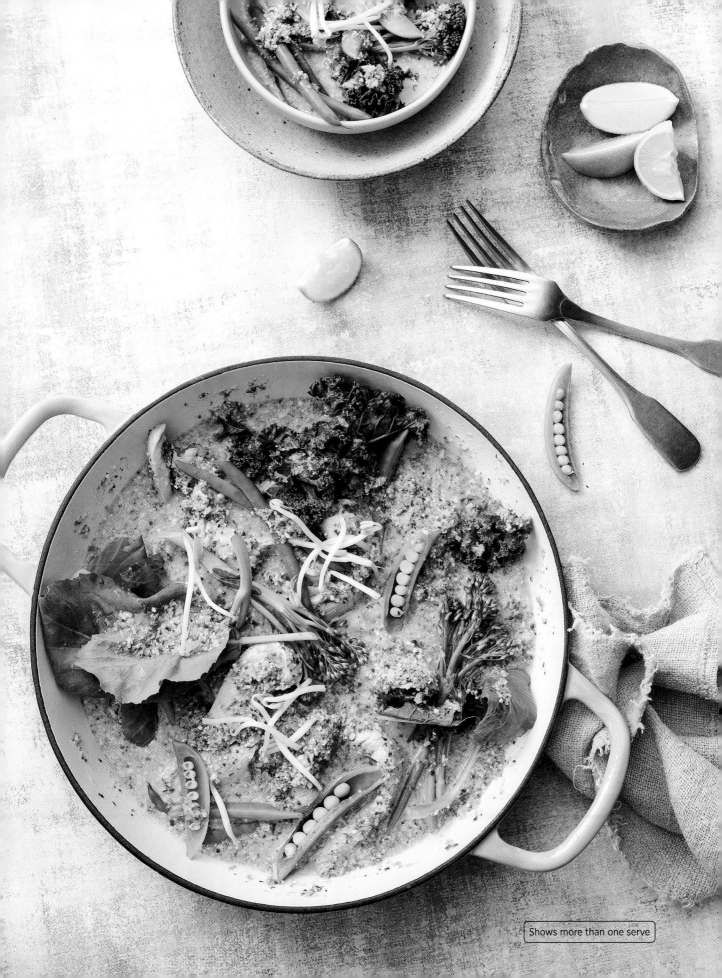

Shows more than one serve

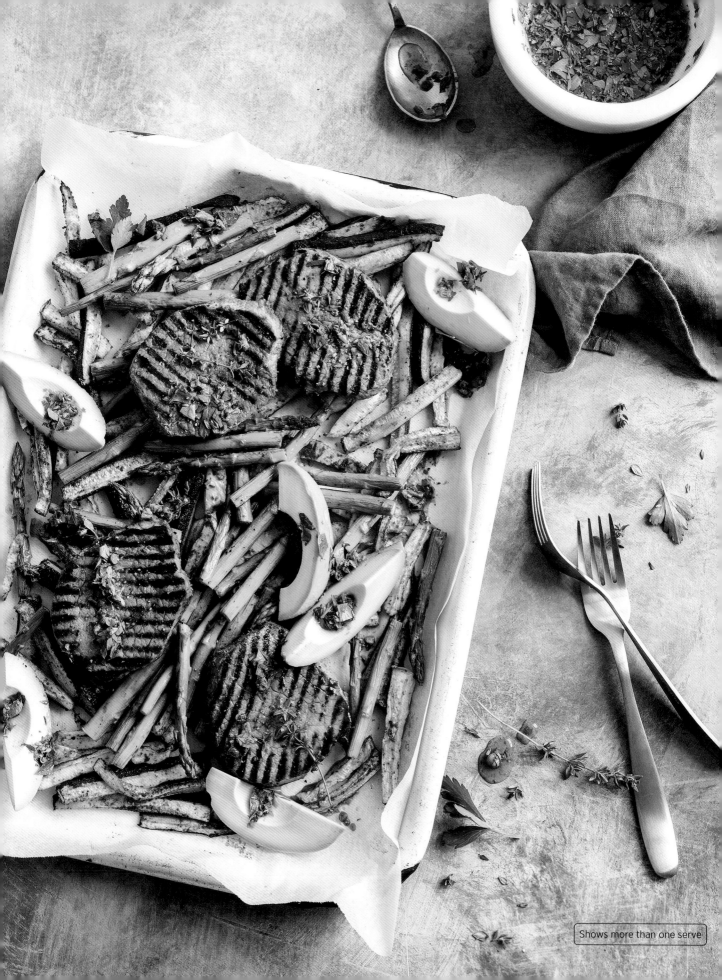

Lean meat, fish, poultry, eggs, tofu: **1.5**
Low–moderate carb vegetables: **4**
Healthy fats: **2**

BBQ steak and vegetable 'fries' with herb sauce

7 G
CARB
PER
SERVE

🍴 **Serves 4**   🕐 **Preparation: 20–25 minutes**
🍲 **Cooking: 40 minutes**   ⓘ **Difficulty: Medium**

300 g peeled celeriac, cut into
   thick matchsticks
300 g zucchini, cut into thick
   matchsticks
1 teaspoon smoked paprika
300 g asparagus, trimmed and
   halved crossways
4 x 150 g beef fillet steaks, excess fat
   and any sinew trimmed
160 g avocado, cut into wedges

HERB SAUCE

½ cup flat-leaf parsley, chopped
2 tablespoons thyme leaves, chopped
1 small clove garlic, crushed
⅓ cup (80 ml) red wine vinegar
1 tablespoon drained capers in brine,
   rinsed and finely chopped

Preheat the oven to 200°C (180°C fan-forced) and line a large baking tray with baking paper.

Toss the celeriac, zucchini and smoked paprika in a large bowl until coated evenly. Season to taste with freshly ground black pepper. Spread the vegetables evenly over the prepared tray and bake for 30 minutes. Add the asparagus to the tray and bake for a further 10 minutes or until all the vegetables are just tender and golden.

Meanwhile, to make the herb sauce, combine all the ingredients in a small bowl. Season to taste with freshly ground black pepper, then cover and chill until required.

Heat a barbecue chargrill to medium–high.

Season the steaks on both sides with freshly ground black pepper. Chargrill for 3 minutes each side for medium or until cooked to your liking. Transfer to a plate, cover loosely with foil and leave to rest for 5 minutes.

Serve the steaks drizzled with any resting juices, with the vegetable 'fries', avocado and the herb sauce.

> **WEEKS 7–12 CARB EXTRAS**
>
> For an extra 9 g carbs per serve, add 200 g (50 g per person) unpeeled sweet potato batons to the baking tray with the celeriac and zucchini.

The recipes in this chapter with 1 unit of lean meat, fish, poultry, eggs and tofu are perfect for lunch, while those with 1.5 units make a great dinner.

MAKE-AHEAD MEALS

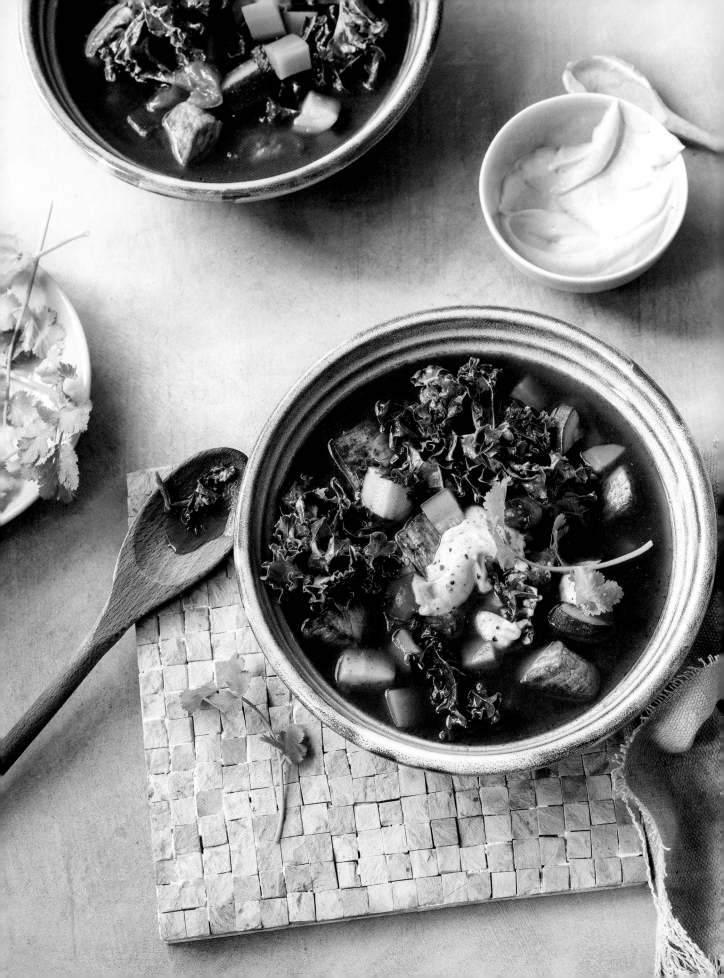

UNITS PER SERVE

Lean meat, fish, poultry, eggs, tofu: **1**
Low–moderate carb vegetables: **2**
Healthy fats: **3**

1 tablespoon olive oil
400 g lean beef eye fillet,
   cut into 2 cm pieces
2 teaspoons curry powder
½ teaspoon ground cinnamon
1 tablespoon salt-reduced tomato paste
75 g cherry tomatoes, halved
150 g carrot, cut into 2 cm pieces
150 g zucchini, cut into 2 cm pieces
1 litre salt-reduced beef stock
75 g torn kale leaves
⅔ cup (160 g) hummus
1 cup coriander sprigs

Hearty spiced beef and vegetable soup with kale

10 G CARB PER SERVE

🍴 **Serves 4**   🕐 **Preparation: 15–20 minutes**
🍲 **Cooking: 20 minutes**   👨‍🍳 **Difficulty: Easy**

Heat the olive oil in a large saucepan over high heat. Add the beef in two batches and cook for 2 minutes each until golden. Transfer to a bowl and cover to keep warm.

Reduce the heat to medium, add the curry powder, cinnamon, tomato paste, tomatoes, carrot and zucchini to the pan and cook, stirring, for 2 minutes or until fragrant. Add the stock and cook, partially covered and stirring occasionally, for 10 minutes or until the liquid has reduced slightly.

Remove from the heat. Return the beef and any juices to the pan and stir in the kale until it has wilted. Season to taste with freshly ground black pepper, then serve topped with hummus and coriander.

WEEKS 7–12 CARB EXTRAS

For an extra 6 g carbs per serve, add 160 g (40 g per person) drained and rinsed tinned chickpeas to the soup before serving.

Note: Ladle the cooled soup into airtight containers and store in the refrigerator for up to 2 days or freeze for up to 3 months. Thaw in the refrigerator overnight, then reheat and serve.

Beef and mushroom stroganoff with garlic spinach and beans

UNITS PER SERVE
Lean meat, fish, poultry, eggs, tofu: **1.5**
Low–moderate carb vegetables: **3**
Healthy fats: **3**

🍴 **Serves 4** 🕐 **Preparation: 25–30 minutes, plus resting time**
🍲 **Cooking: 25 minutes** 🍳 **Difficulty: Easy**

2 tablespoons olive oil
600 g lean beef rump steak, cut into
  2 cm pieces
1 red onion (150 g), cut into thin wedges
2 cloves garlic, crushed
400 g button mushrooms, thickly sliced
1 teaspoon sweet paprika
1 tablespoon salt-reduced tomato paste
2 teaspoons Dijon mustard
1 tablespoon Worcestershire sauce
2 fresh bay leaves (see notes)
2 cups (500 ml) salt-reduced beef stock
50 g natural Greek-style yoghurt

GARLIC SPINACH AND BEANS

1 tablespoon olive oil
2 cloves garlic, crushed
200 g baby spinach leaves
300 g green beans, halved diagonally
¼ cup chopped flat-leaf parsley

Heat the olive oil in a large deep frying pan over high heat. Add the beef in three batches and cook for 2 minutes each. Transfer to a bowl and cover to keep warm.

Reduce the heat to medium. Add the onion and cook, stirring occasionally, for 3 minutes or until just starting to soften. Add the garlic, mushrooms, paprika and tomato paste and cook, stirring, for 2 minutes. Add the mustard, Worcestershire sauce, bay leaves and stock and cook, stirring occasionally, for 10 minutes or until the liquid has reduced by half.

Remove from the heat and return the beef and any juices to the pan. Season to taste with freshly ground black pepper, then leave to stand, uncovered, for 10 minutes. Stir through the yoghurt until just combined.

Meanwhile, to make the garlic spinach and beans, heat the olive oil in a large saucepan over high heat. Add the garlic, spinach, beans and ½ cup (125 ml) water and cook, stirring, for 3 minutes or until the spinach has wilted and the beans are just tender. Stir in the parsley and season to taste with freshly ground black pepper.

Serve the stroganoff with the garlic spinach and beans.

WEEKS 7–12 CARB EXTRAS

For an extra 9 g carbs per serve, serve with 200 g (50 g per person) peeled, steamed and mashed sweet potato.

Notes: Spoon the cooled stroganoff and spinach mixture into airtight containers and store in the refrigerator for up to 2 days or freeze for up to 3 months. Thaw in the refrigerator overnight, then reheat and serve.

You can use one dried bay leaf instead of two fresh leaves, if preferred.

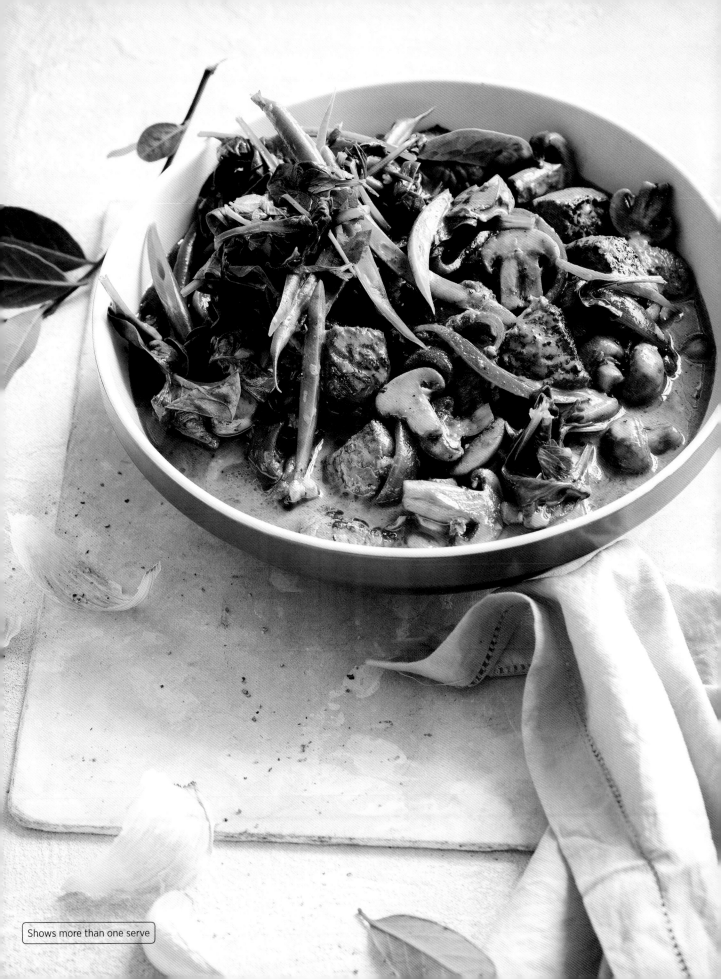

Shows more than one serve

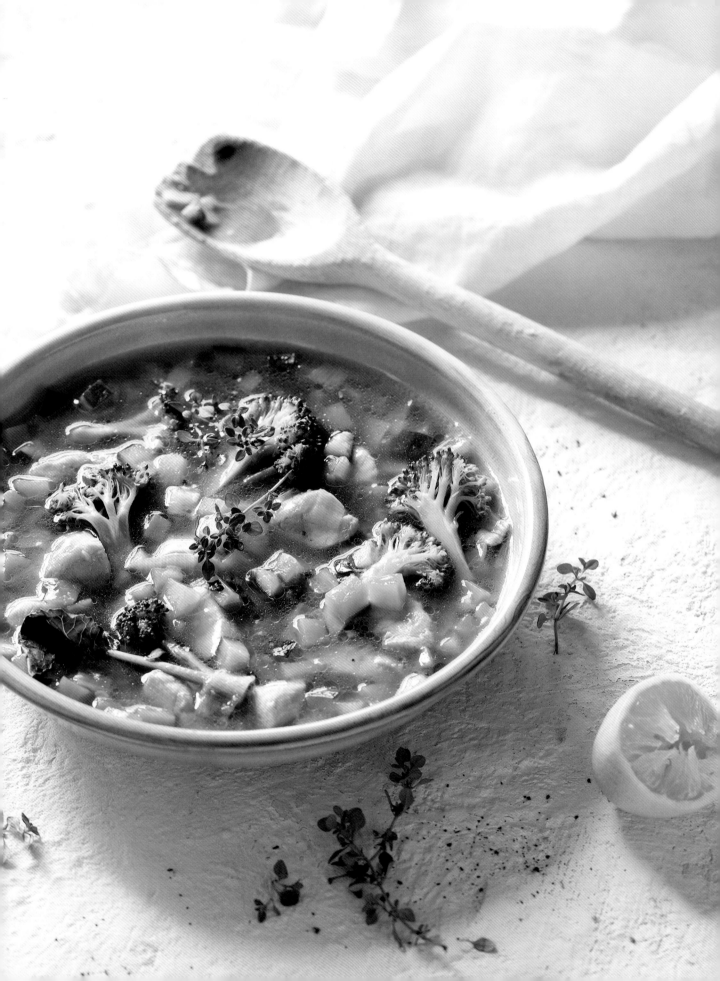

Lean meat, fish, poultry, eggs, tofu: **1.5**
Low–moderate carb vegetables: **3**
Healthy fats: **2**

Lemon and garlic chicken stew

7 G
CARB
PER
SERVE

🍴 **Serves 4**   🕐 **Preparation: 25–30 minutes**
🍲 **Cooking: 25 minutes**   ⏱ **Difficulty: Easy**

2 tablespoons olive oil
4 cloves garlic, sliced
600 g lean chicken
   tenderloins, chopped
150 g carrot, finely chopped
100 g peeled swede, finely chopped
50 g leek, white part only,
   finely chopped
300 g zucchini, finely chopped
2 cups (500 ml) salt-reduced
   chicken stock
1 tablespoon lemon thyme leaves
300 g broccoli florets
juice of 2 lemons

Heat the olive oil in a large saucepan over medium–high heat. Add the garlic and chicken and cook, stirring occasionally, for 5 minutes or until light golden. Add the carrot, swede, leek and zucchini and cook, stirring occasionally, for 3 minutes or until the leek is starting to soften.

Add the stock and lemon thyme and cook, partially covered and stirring occasionally, for 15 minutes or until cooked and the liquid has reduced by half. Add the broccoli and cook, covered, for 2 minutes.

Remove the pan from the heat and stir in the lemon juice. Season to taste with freshly ground black pepper and serve.

WEEKS 7–12 CARB EXTRAS

For an extra 8 g carbs per serve, serve with 200 g (50 g per person) cooked quinoa.

Note: Spoon the cooled stew into airtight containers and store in the refrigerator for up to 2 days or freeze for up to 3 months. Thaw in the refrigerator overnight, then reheat and serve.

Broccolini fish parcels with saffron pine nuts

UNITS PER SERVE

Lean meat, fish, poultry, eggs, tofu: **1.5**
Low–moderate carb vegetables: **3**
Healthy fats: **4**

🍴 **Serves 4**   🕐 **Preparation: 30–35 minutes**
🍳 **Cooking: 25 minutes**   ⓘ **Difficulty: Easy**

150 g English spinach leaves
1 lemon, sliced into rounds
75 g celery stalk, thinly sliced
½ (75 g) red onion, cut into thin wedges
100 g carrot, cut into thin matchsticks
150 g tomato, chopped
150 g broccolini, trimmed, halved
    lengthways and cut into 5 cm lengths
150 g yellow squash, thinly sliced
    into rounds
4 x 150 g barramundi fillets, skin on
    and pin-boned
2 tablespoons dill

SAFFRON SPREAD

60 g olive oil margarine
2 cloves garlic, crushed
1 teaspoon saffron threads
40 g pine nuts, toasted and chopped

Preheat the oven to 200°C (180°C fan-forced). Place a large baking tray in the oven to heat through.

Tear off four large pieces of foil and place on a work surface. Top each piece with a large piece of baking paper.

Place the spinach in the centre of the paper and foil wrappers. Top with lemon slices, then the celery, onion, carrot, tomato, broccolini and squash. Rest the barramundi fillets on top and season to taste with freshly ground black pepper.

To make the saffron spread, combine all the ingredients in a small bowl. Season to taste with freshly ground black pepper, then spread evenly over the barramundi.

Sprinkle over the dill, then fold in the ends of the paper and foil and wrap up tightly to form neat, airtight parcels. Carefully transfer the parcels to the baking tray in the oven and bake for 25 minutes or until the vegetables and fish are tender. Serve immediately.

> **WEEKS 7–12 CARB EXTRAS**
>
> For an extra 9 g carbs per serve, serve with 160 g (40 g per person) cooked puy lentils.

Note: You can freeze the uncooked parcels in airtight containers for up to 3 months. Thaw in the refrigerator overnight and bake as directed.

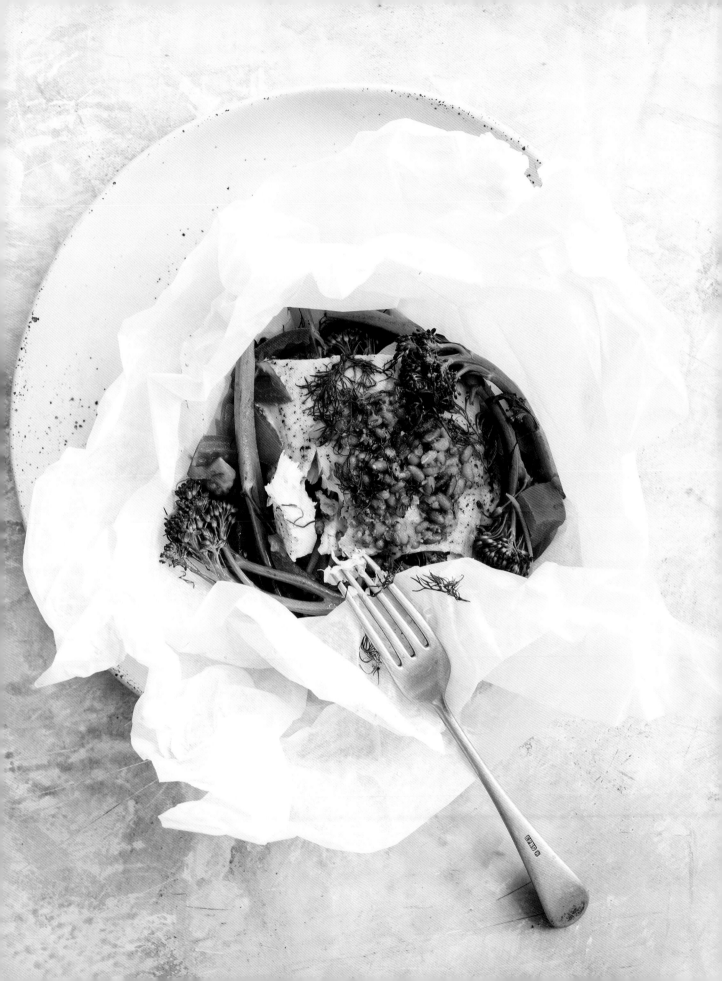

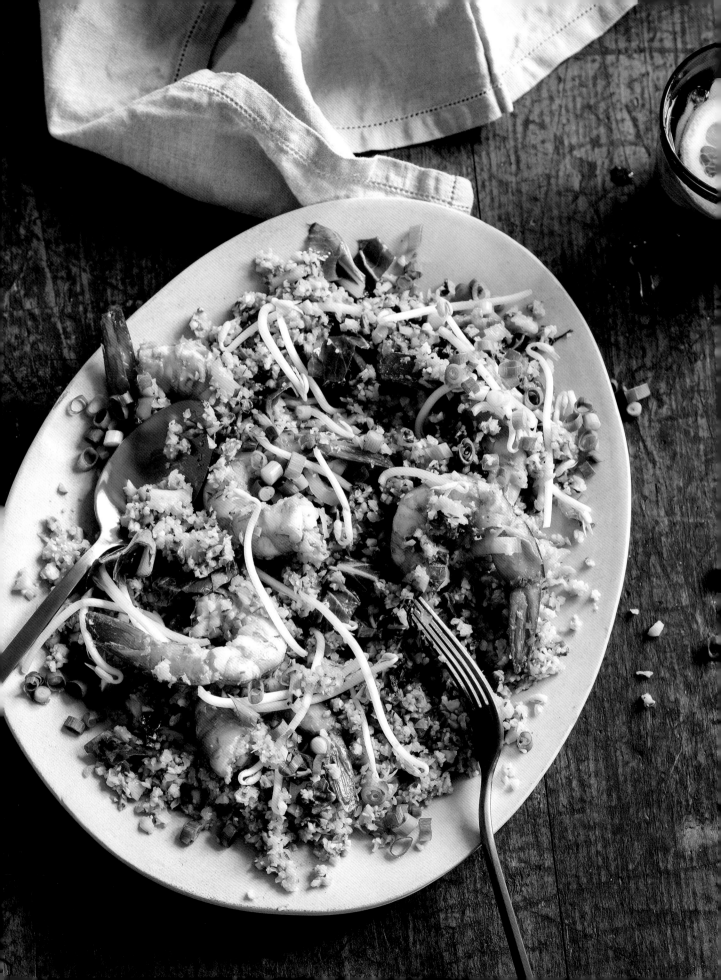

UNITS PER SERVE

Lean meat, fish, poultry, eggs, tofu: **1.5**
Low–moderate carb vegetables: **3**
Healthy fats: **2**

Prawn and zucchini fried 'rice'

5 G CARB PER SERVE

🍴 **Serves 4**   🕐 **Preparation: 20–25 minutes**
🍳 **Cooking: 10 minutes**   👩‍🍳 **Difficulty: Easy**

300 g zucchini, chopped
225 g cauliflower florets
2 tablespoons rice bran oil
2 stalks lemongrass, white part only,
    finely chopped
2 cloves garlic, crushed
1 small fresh red chilli, finely chopped
600 g peeled, deveined raw king
    prawns, tails left on
225 g pak choy, shredded
¼ cup (60 ml) salt-reduced soy sauce
4 spring onions, thinly sliced
75 g bean sprouts, trimmed

Process the zucchini and cauliflower separately in a food processor until they resemble rice grains.

Heat the rice bran oil in a large wok over high heat, add the lemongrass, garlic, chilli and prawns and stir-fry for 5 minutes or until cooked and golden. Add the pak choy and soy sauce and stir-fry for 1 minute or until the pak choy is just starting to wilt. Add the zucchini and cauliflower rice and stir-fry for 1 minute.

Remove the wok from the heat. Toss through the spring onion and sprouts, and serve.

WEEKS 7–12 CARB EXTRAS

For an extra 8 g carbs per serve, toss through 200 g (50 g per person) cooked quinoa with the spring onion and sprouts before serving.

Note: Store the cooled mixture in airtight containers in the refrigerator for up to 2 days or freeze for up to 3 months. Thaw in the refrigerator overnight, then reheat in the wok and serve.

UNITS PER SERVE
Lean meat, fish, poultry, eggs, tofu: **1.5**
Low–moderate carb vegetables: **3**
Healthy fats: **3**

Mustard and tarragon chicken with grilled veg

8 G CARB PER SERVE

🍴 **Serves 4** 🕐 **Preparation: 15–30 minutes, plus marinating time**
🍳 **Cooking: 15 minutes** 👨‍🍳 **Difficulty: Easy**

600 g lean chicken tenderloins
2 tablespoons red wine vinegar
¼ cup tarragon leaves
1 tablespoon wholegrain mustard
1 tablespoon extra virgin olive oil
1 red onion (150 g), thinly sliced
   into rounds
300 g asparagus, trimmed
300 g zucchini, cut into matchsticks
⅔ cup (160 g) hummus
½ teaspoon smoked paprika
⅓ cup basil leaves

Combine the chicken, vinegar, tarragon, mustard and olive oil in a glass or ceramic bowl. Cover and marinate in the refrigerator for 20 minutes.

Preheat the oven grill to high. Place a large baking tray under the grill to preheat.

Carefully add the onion, asparagus and zucchini to the hot tray. Top with the chicken mixture and grill for 12 minutes or until cooked and golden.

Spoon the hummus evenly onto serving plates and sprinkle with the paprika. Top with the grilled chicken and vegetables, scatter the basil over and serve.

WEEKS 7–12 CARB EXTRAS

For an extra 8 g carbs per serve, add 480 g (120 g per person) baby green peas to the tray when cooking the chicken mixture.

Note: Store the uncooked marinated chicken mixture in airtight containers in the refrigerator for up to 2 days or freeze for up to 6 months. Thaw in the refrigerator overnight, then cook as instructed in the recipe.

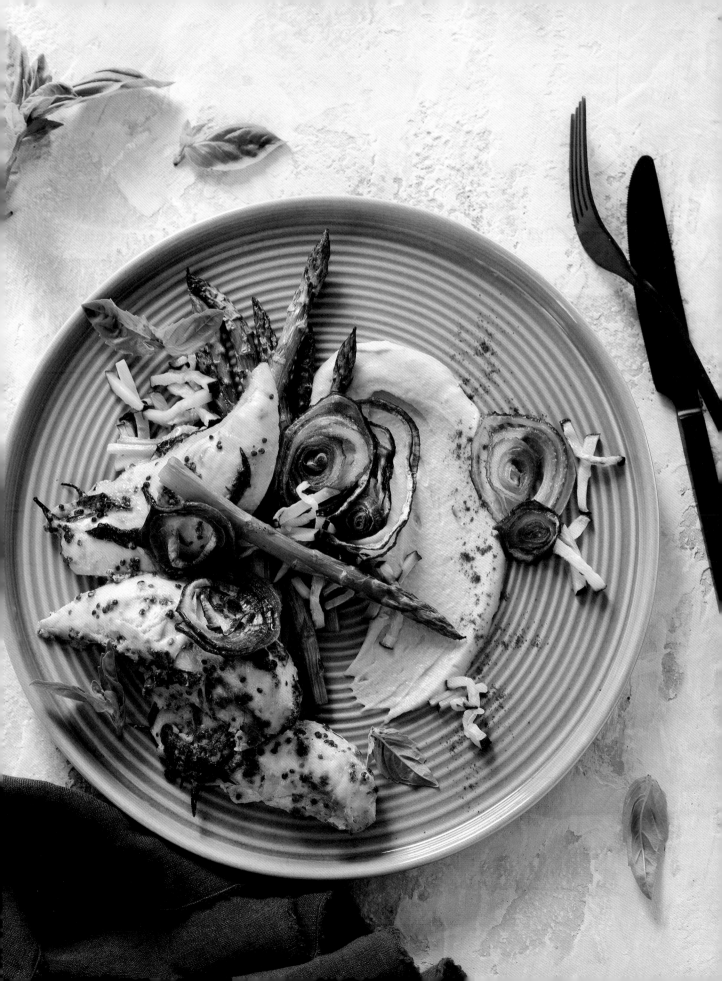

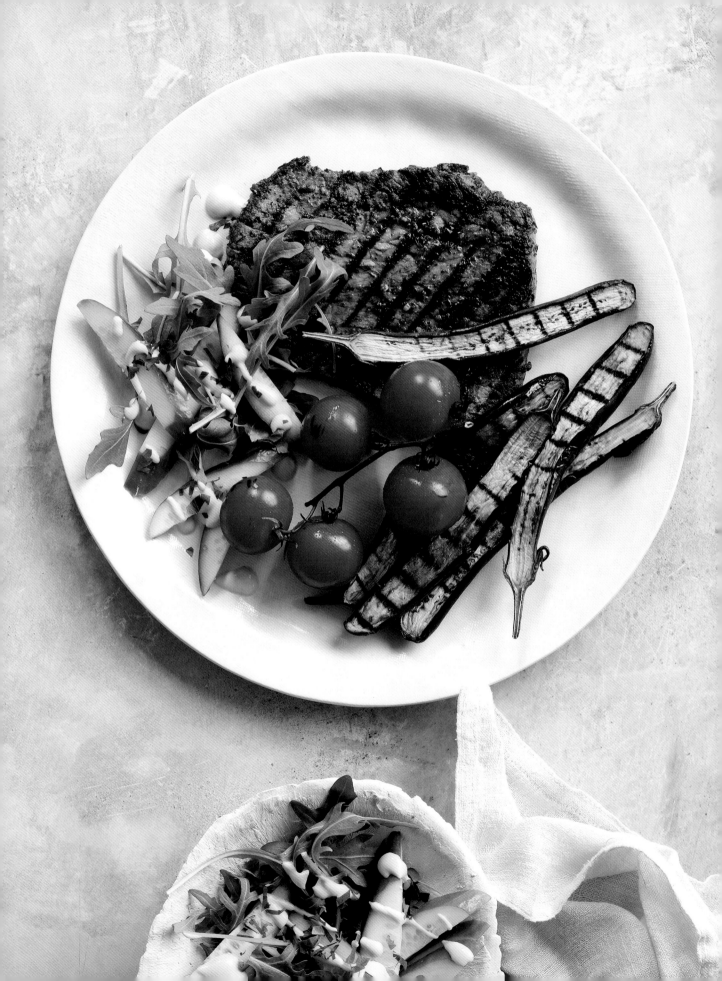

Lean meat, fish, poultry, eggs, tofu: **1.5**
Low–moderate carb vegetables: **2.5**
Healthy fats: **4**

2 tablespoons olive oil
1 tablespoon dried harissa spice mix
1 tablespoon chopped oregano
1 tablespoon freshly ground
    black pepper
4 x 150 g portions beef topside
300 g baby eggplants,
    halved lengthways
250 g cherry tomatoes

TAHINI CUCUMBER
2 tablespoons tahini
¼ cup (60 ml) red wine vinegar
300 g Lebanese cucumbers, halved
    lengthways, thinly sliced diagonally
¼ cup chopped flat-leaf parsley
50 g rocket leaves

Harissa-marinated beef with chargrilled eggplant and tomatoes

8 G
CARB
PER
SERVE

🍴 **Serves 4**   🕐 **Preparation: 15–30 minutes, plus marinating time**
🍲 **Cooking: 15 minutes**   🍶 **Difficulty: Easy**

Combine the olive oil, spice mix, oregano, pepper and beef in a glass or ceramic bowl. Cover and marinate in the refrigerator for 20 minutes.

To make the tahini cucumber, place the tahini and vinegar in a small bowl and whisk with a fork, adding 1–2 tablespoons water if the mixture is a little thick. In a separate bowl, toss the cucumber, parsley and rocket. Chill separately until required.

Heat a large chargrill pan over high heat. Add the eggplant and tomatoes and cook, turning once, for 5 minutes or until just tender and golden. Divide among serving plates.

Cook the beef on the chargrill for 3 minutes each side for medium or until cooked to your liking. Add to the serving plates, then cover loosely with foil and rest for 5 minutes.

Arrange the steak, eggplant and tomatoes on serving plates. Add the cucumber salad, drizzle it with the tahini dressing and serve.

WEEKS 7–12 CARB EXTRAS

For an extra 6 g carbs per serve, add 160 g (40 g per person) drained and rinsed tinned chickpeas to the tahini cucumber.

Note: Store the uncooked marinated beef mixture in airtight containers in the refrigerator for up to 2 days or freeze for up to 6 months. Thaw in the refrigerator overnight, then cook as instructed. The tahini cucumber is best prepared close to serving time.

UNITS PER SERVE
Lean meat, fish, poultry, eggs, tofu: **1.5**
Low–moderate carb vegetables: **3**
Healthy fats: **3**

Sesame-spiced salmon with snowpea salad

10 G CARB PER SERVE

🍴 **Serves 4**   🕐 **Preparation: 20–25 minutes, plus marinating time**
🍲 **Cooking: 5 minutes**   👨‍🍳 **Difficulty: Easy**

¼ cup (60 ml) oyster sauce

1 teaspoon sesame oil

2 tablespoons sesame seeds

1 fresh long red chilli,
    thinly sliced diagonally

5 cm piece ginger, cut into
    long thin strips

¼ cup (60 ml) apple cider vinegar

4 x 150 g salmon fillets, skin on
    and pin-boned

150 g Chinese broccoli, trimmed

300 g snow peas

150 g zucchini, cut with a vegetable
    peeler into long thin ribbons

4 spring onions, thinly sliced diagonally

160 g avocado, sliced

lime wedges, to serve

Combine the oyster sauce, sesame oil, sesame seeds, chilli, ginger, 1 tablespoon of the vinegar and the salmon in a glass or ceramic bowl. Cover and marinate in the refrigerator for 20 minutes.

Preheat the oven grill to high.

Place the salmon, skin-side down, on a baking tray and spoon over the marinade. Cook under the grill for 5 minutes for medium or until cooked to your liking. Transfer to a plate and cover to keep warm.

Meanwhile, place the Chinese broccoli and snow peas in a heatproof bowl. Cover with boiling water, and stand for 1 minute or until the broccoli is just wilted. Drain and refresh under cold running water. Return to the bowl. Add the zucchini, spring onion, avocado and remaining vinegar and gently toss to combine.

Divide the zucchini mixture among serving plates. Top with the salmon and serve with lime wedges.

WEEKS 7–12 CARB EXTRAS

For an extra 8 g carbs per serve, add 480 g (120 g per person) thawed green peas to the zucchini mixture.

Note: Store the uncooked marinated salmon mixture in airtight containers in the refrigerator for up to 2 days or freeze for up to 6 months. Thaw in the refrigerator overnight before cooking as instructed.

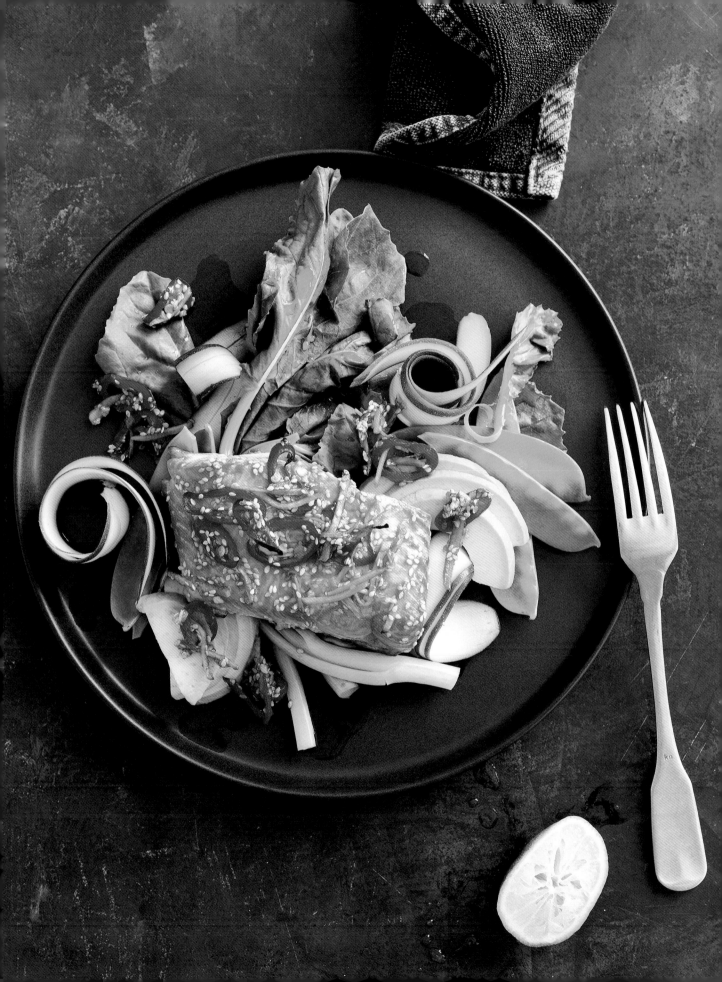

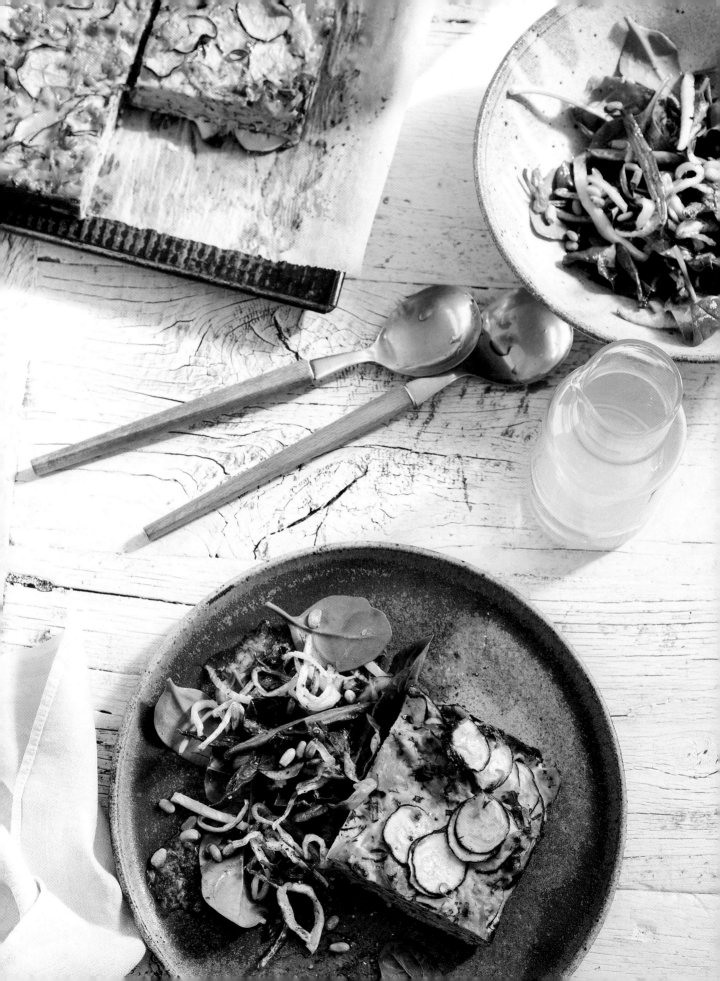

Tuna and zucchini bake with lemony greens

UNITS PER SERVE

Lean meat, fish, poultry, eggs, tofu: **1.5**
Dairy and dairy alternatives: **1**
Low–moderate carb vegetables: **3**
Healthy fats: **4**

🍴 **Serves 4** 🕐 **Preparation: 25–30 minutes, plus resting time**
🍲 **Cooking: 30 minutes** 🍳 **Difficulty: Easy**

1 x 425 g tin tuna in springwater,
   drained and flaked
4 eggs
450 g zucchini, very thinly sliced
   into rounds
4 spring onions, very thinly sliced
110 g ricotta
40 g cheddar, finely grated
½ cup dill
¼ cup chopped chives

LEMONY GREENS

2 tablespoons olive oil
25 g green beans, trimmed and
   halved diagonally
100 g peeled celeriac, cut into
   long thin strips
50 g baby spinach leaves
finely grated zest and juice of 1 lemon
80 g pine nuts, toasted

Preheat the oven to 200°C (180°C fan-forced). Line the base and sides of a 4 cm deep, 28 cm x 18 cm baking dish with baking paper.

Combine the tuna, eggs, zucchini, spring onion, ricotta, cheddar, dill and chives in a large bowl. Season to taste with freshly ground black pepper. Spoon the mixture into the prepared tin and level the surface. Bake for 30 minutes or until golden and cooked through. Rest for 5 minutes in the tin before slicing.

Meanwhile, to make the lemony greens, heat the olive oil in a large deep frying pan over medium–high heat. Add the beans and celeriac and cook, stirring occasionally, for 10 minutes or until cooked and golden. Stir in the spinach, lemon zest and lemon juice and cook until wilted. Remove the pan from the heat and stir in the pine nuts. Season to taste with freshly ground black pepper.

Serve the tuna bake with the lemony greens.

WEEKS 7-12 CARB EXTRAS

For an extra 7 g carbs per serve, serve with 2 (½ per person) wholemeal pita breads.

Note: Store the cooled tuna bake in airtight containers in the refrigerator for up to 2 days or freeze for up to 3 months. Thaw in the refrigerator overnight before reheating to serve. Prepare the lemony greens close to serving time.

Use 100 g very finely sliced carrot in place of the celeriac, if preferred.

Lean meat, fish, poultry, eggs, tofu: **1**
Low–moderate carb vegetables: **2**
Healthy fats: **5**

Chicken, silverbeet and lentil dhal

8 G CARB PER SERVE

🍴 **Serves 4**   🕐 **Preparation: 20–25 minutes**
🍲 **Cooking: 30 minutes**   🎩 **Difficulty: Easy**

1 tablespoon rice bran oil
400 g lean chicken tenderloins, chopped
2 teaspoons ground turmeric
1 teaspoon garam masala
2 cm piece ginger, finely grated
1 clove garlic, crushed
300 g tomatoes, finely chopped
150 g zucchini, finely chopped
150 g carrot, finely chopped
320 g drained and rinsed tinned lentils
1 litre salt-reduced chicken stock
150 g silverbeet leaves, white stalks removed, shredded
lime wedges, to serve

ALMOND SPRINKLE

120 g slivered almonds, toasted
¼ cup coriander sprigs
2 tablespoons chopped flat-leaf parsley

Heat the rice bran oil in a large saucepan over high heat. Add the chicken, turmeric, garam masala, ginger, garlic and tomato and cook, stirring occasionally, for 10 minutes or until the chicken is golden and the tomato has collapsed.

Add the zucchini, carrot, lentils and stock. Cook, stirring occasionally, for 20 minutes or until the lentils are mushy and the stock has reduced by two-thirds. Stir in the silverbeet until wilted. Season to taste with freshly ground black pepper.

To make the almond sprinkle, combine all the ingredients in a small bowl. Season to taste with freshly ground black pepper.

Ladle the dhal into shallow bowls, top with the almond sprinkle and serve with lime wedges.

WEEKS 7–12 CARB EXTRAS

For an extra 9 g carbs per serve, add an additional 160 g (40 g per person) rinsed tinned lentils with the zucchini and carrot.

Note: Store the cooled dhal mixture in airtight containers in the refrigerator for up to 2 days or freeze for up to 3 months. Thaw in the refrigerator overnight before reheating to serve.

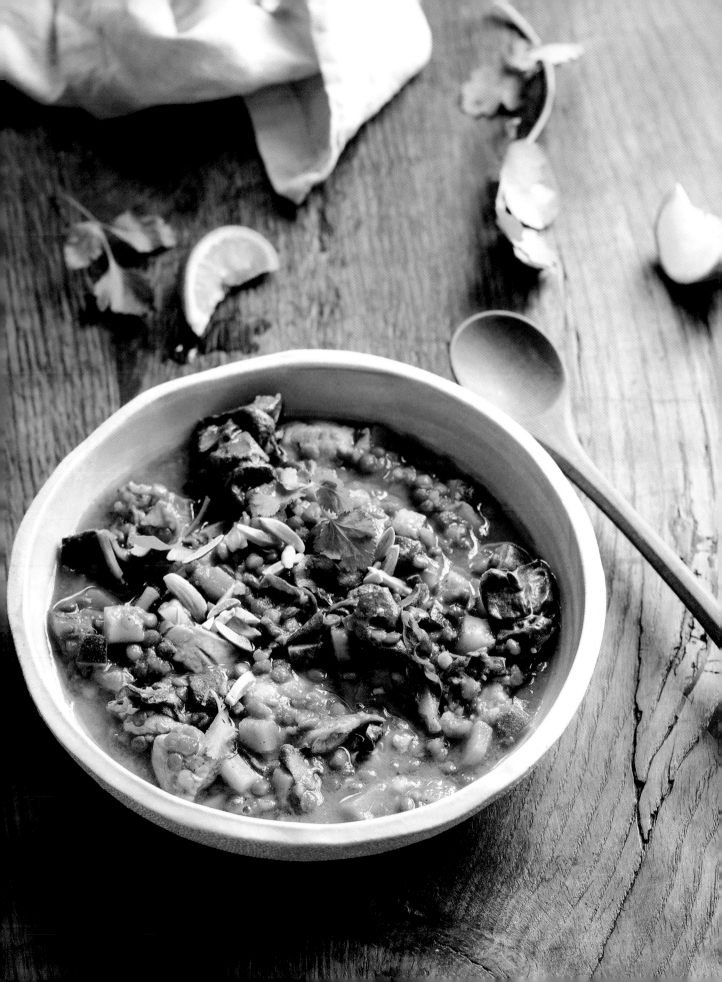

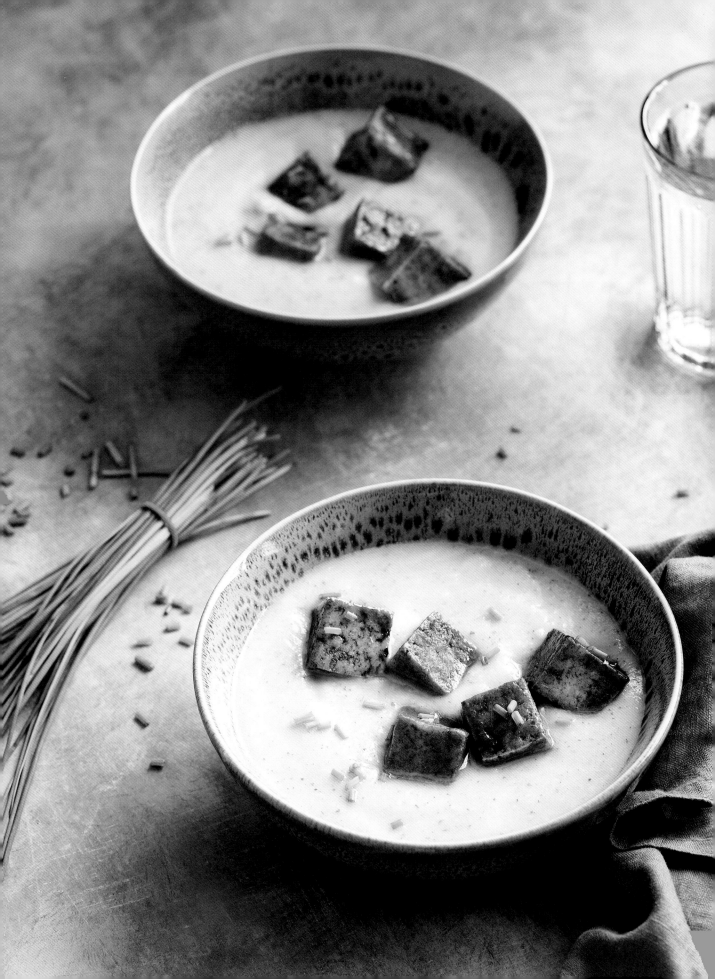

UNITS PER SERVE

Lean meat, fish, poultry, eggs, tofu: **1**
Dairy and dairy alternatives: **0.5**
Low-moderate carb vegetables: **3**
Healthy fats: **4**

300 g peeled celeriac, chopped
300 g zucchini, sliced
2 tablespoons thyme leaves
2 teaspoons chopped rosemary
1 litre salt-reduced vegetable stock
110 g cottage cheese
160 g avocado, chopped

BALSAMIC TOFU CROUTONS

2 tablespoons olive oil
400 g firm tofu, cut into cubes
2 tablespoons balsamic vinegar
2 tablespoons chopped chives

Creamy celeriac soup with balsamic tofu croutons

🍴 **Serves 4**　🕐 **Preparation: 25–30 minutes, plus standing time**
🍲 **Cooking: 20 minutes**　🥄 **Difficulty: Easy**

To make the balsamic tofu croutons, heat the olive oil in a large frying pan over high heat, add the tofu and cook, stirring, for 5 minutes or until crisp and golden. Add the balsamic and immediately shake the pan to coat the tofu (the vinegar will bubble and reduce very quickly). Remove the pan from the heat. Stir through the chives and season to taste with freshly ground black pepper. Set aside until required.

Place the celeriac, zucchini, thyme, rosemary and stock in a large saucepan over medium–high heat. Cook, partially covered and stirring occasionally, for 15 minutes or until the vegetables are tender.

Remove the pan from the heat and leave to stand for 10 minutes. Stir in the cottage cheese and avocado and season to taste with freshly ground black pepper. Using a stick blender, blend the mixture together until very smooth. Divide the soup among serving bowls and top with the balsamic tofu croutons.

WEEKS 7–12 CARB EXTRAS

For an extra 7 g carbs per serve, add 200 g (50 g per person) drained and rinsed tinned cannellini beans to the soup just before serving to heat through.

Note: Store the cooled soup and tofu mixtures in airtight containers in the refrigerator for up to 2 days or freeze for up to 3 months. Thaw in the refrigerator overnight before reheating to serve.

Lean meat, fish, poultry, eggs, tofu: **1.5**
Low–moderate carb vegetables: **3**
Healthy fats: **3**

Chilli beef and mushroom stir-fry

4 G CARB PER SERVE

🍴 **Serves 4** 🕐 **Preparation: 20–25 minutes**
🍲 **Cooking: 10 minutes** 🎲 **Difficulty: Easy**

2 tablespoons rice bran oil

2 fresh long red chillies, thinly
sliced diagonally

600 g lean beef eye fillet, thinly sliced

450 g mixed Asian mushrooms (enoki,
oyster, shiitake)

150 g broccoli florets

150 g baby bok choy,
halved lengthways

2 tablespoons Shaoxing rice wine
or dry sherry

1 tablespoon oyster sauce

3 cm piece ginger, finely grated

½ cup (125 ml) salt-reduced beef stock

80 g macadamias, toasted and
finely chopped

Heat 2 teaspoons of the rice bran oil in a large wok over high heat.
Add the chilli and stir-fry for 2 minutes or until crisp and golden.
Remove with a slotted spoon and place in a large bowl.

Heat the remaining oil in the same wok over high heat. Add the beef
in batches and stir-fry for 2 minutes or until golden. Transfer to the
bowl with the chilli and cover to keep warm.

Add the mushrooms, broccoli, bok choy, rice wine, oyster sauce, ginger
and stock to the wok and stir-fry for 2 minutes or until the vegetables
are just tender and the greens start to wilt. Return the beef mixture
and any juices to the wok and toss to combine.

Remove the wok from the heat and toss through the macadamias.
Season to taste with freshly ground black pepper and serve.

> **WEEKS 7–12 CARB EXTRAS**
>
> For an extra 7 g carbs per serve, serve with 2 (½ per person)
> wholemeal pita breads.

Note: Store the cooled stir-fry mixture in airtight containers in
the refrigerator for up to 2 days or freeze for up to 3 months.
Thaw in the refrigerator overnight before reheating to serve.

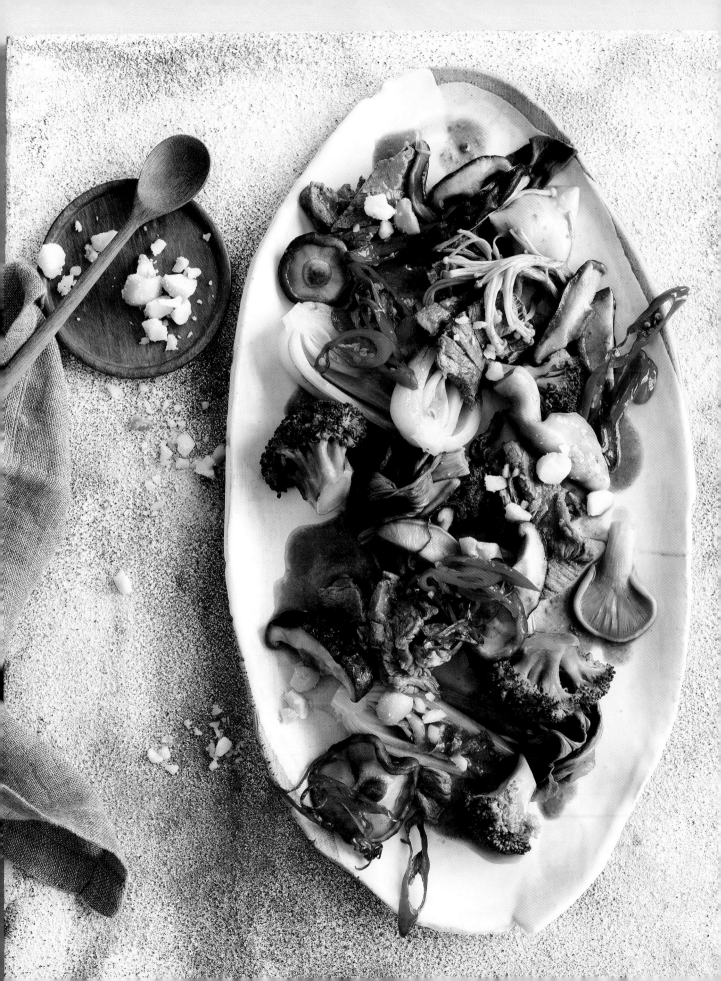

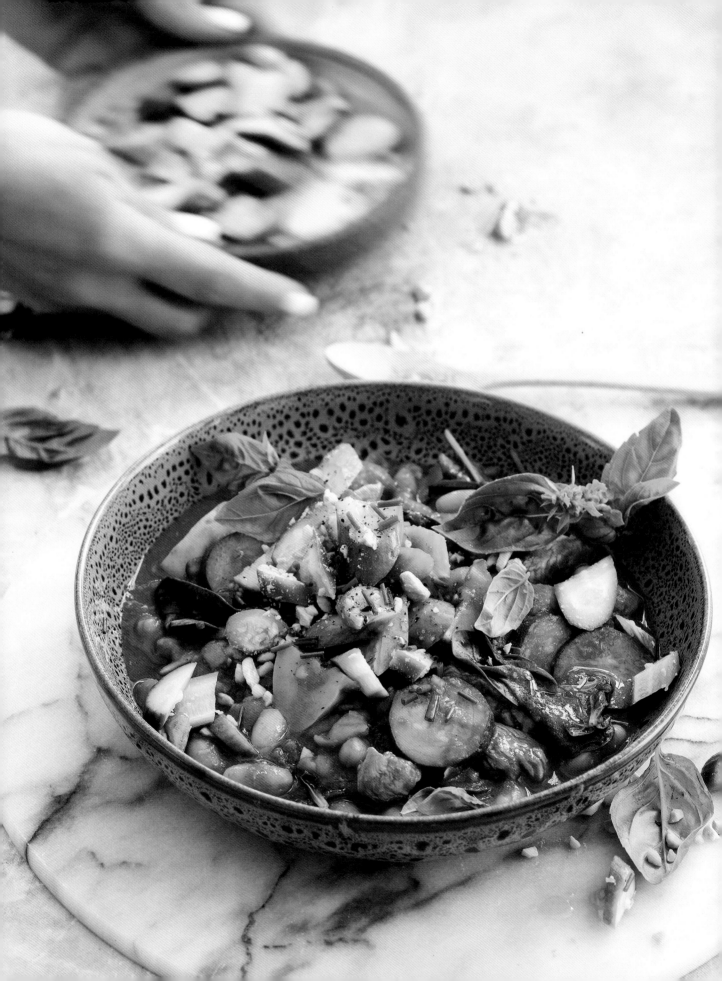

Lean meat, fish, poultry, eggs, tofu: **1**
Breads, cereals, legumes, starchy
vegetables: **0.5**
Low-moderate carb vegetables: **3**
Healthy fats: **5**

---

1 tablespoon olive oil
400 g lean chicken breast fillets,
thinly sliced
2 teaspoons sweet paprika
2 cloves garlic, crushed
150 g zucchini, sliced into rounds
200 g yellow squash, quartered
1 cup (250 ml) tomato passata
200 g drained and rinsed tinned
cannellini beans
100 g baby spinach leaves
1 cup basil leaves

CUCUMBER AND ALMOND SALSA

150 g baby cucumbers,
finely chopped
120 g whole natural almonds,
toasted and chopped
2 tablespoons chopped chives
2 tablespoons red wine vinegar
1 tablespoon extra virgin olive oil

Chicken and cannellini ragu with cucumber and almond salsa

🍴 Serves 4   🕐 Preparation: 20–25 minutes
🍲 Cooking: 30 minutes   ☺ Difficulty: Easy

To make the cucumber and almond salsa, combine all the ingredients in a bowl and season to taste with freshly ground black pepper. Set aside until required.

Heat the olive oil in a large saucepan over high heat. Add the chicken, paprika and garlic and cook, stirring occasionally, for 5 minutes or until the chicken is starting to brown.

Reduce the heat to medium–low. Add the zucchini, squash, passata, cannellini beans and 1 cup (250 ml) water and cook, partially covered and stirring occasionally, for 25 minutes or until cooked and the sauce has reduced by half. Stir in the spinach until it wilts, then remove the pan from the heat. Stir in the basil and season to taste with freshly ground black pepper.

Spoon the ragu into shallow bowls and serve topped with the cucumber and almond salsa.

> **WEEKS 7–12 CARB EXTRAS**
>
> For an extra 6–8 g carbs per serve, serve with 200 g (50 g per person) cooked quinoa or 2 slices (½ slice per person) toasted mixed grain bread.

Note: Store the cooled ragu mixture in airtight containers in the refrigerator for up to 2 days or freeze for up to 3 months. Thaw in the refrigerator overnight before reheating to serve.

Lean meat, fish, poultry, eggs, tofu: **1.5**
Low–moderate carb vegetables: **2.5**
Healthy fats: **3**

Pork patties with carrot and swede mash

7 G CARB PER SERVE

🍴 **Serves 4**   🕐 **Preparation: 30–35 minutes, plus refrigerating time**
🥘 **Cooking: 15 minutes**   👨‍🍳 **Difficulty: Easy**

600 g lean pork tenderloin, sinew removed, chopped
½ cup flat-leaf parsley leaves, plus extra finely chopped leaves to serve
3 teaspoons cumin seeds
1 tablespoon wholegrain mustard
2 tablespoons olive oil
finely grated lemon zest, to serve

CARROT AND SWEDE MASH

150 g carrot, chopped
150 g peeled swede, finely chopped
300 g peeled celeriac, chopped
80 g avocado
finely grated zest and juice of ½ lemon

Process the pork in a food processor until minced. Add the parsley, cumin seeds and mustard and process until well combined, smooth and sticky. Season to taste with freshly ground black pepper. Using slightly damp hands, divide the mixture into eight equal portions and form into smooth patties. Transfer to a baking tray lined with baking paper. Cover and chill for 15 minutes to set firm.

To make the carrot and swede mash, steam the carrot, swede and celeriac for 15 minutes or until tender. Transfer to a bowl. Add the avocado, lemon zest and juice, and mash together until well combined. Season to taste with freshly ground black pepper. Cover to keep warm.

Meanwhile, heat the olive oil in a large frying pan over medium–high heat. Cook the patties, turning occasionally, for 15 minutes or until cooked through and golden.

Serve the pork patties with the carrot and swede mash, topped with extra parsley and lemon zest.

> **WEEKS 7–12 CARB EXTRAS**
>
> For an extra 9 g carbs per serve, steam 200 g (50 g per person) peeled, chopped sweet potato with the other vegetables when making the mash.

Note: For the mash, you can use the same amount of zucchini in place of the celeriac if preferred; it will result in a slightly different texture but will be just as delicious.

Store the cooled patties and the mash mixture in airtight containers in the refrigerator for up to 2 days or freeze them for up to 3 months. Thaw in the refrigerator overnight before reheating to serve.

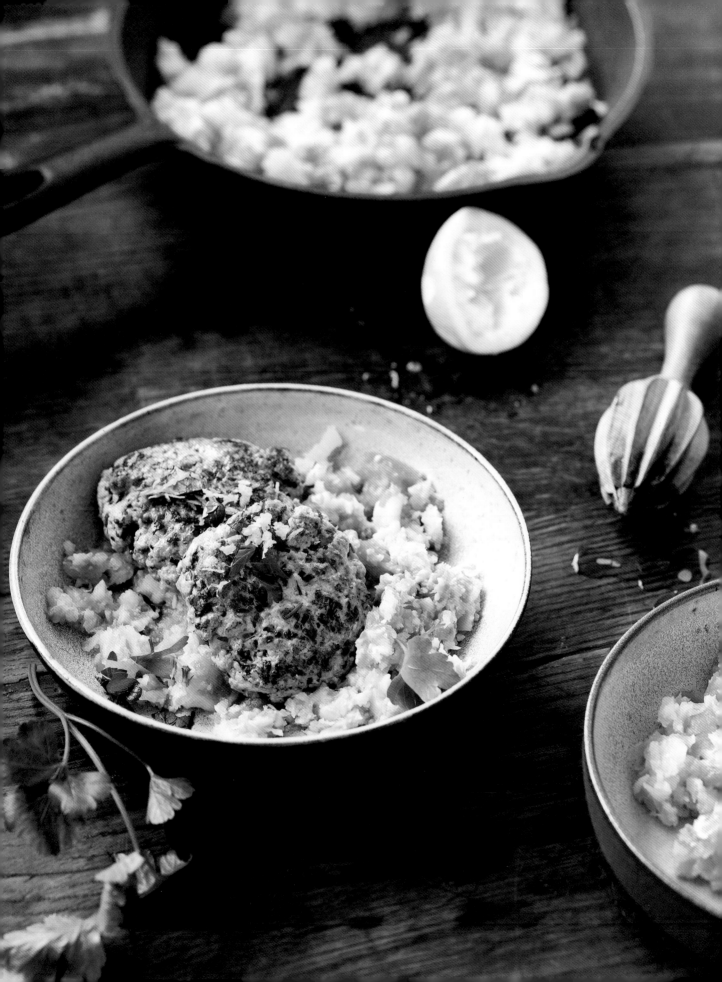

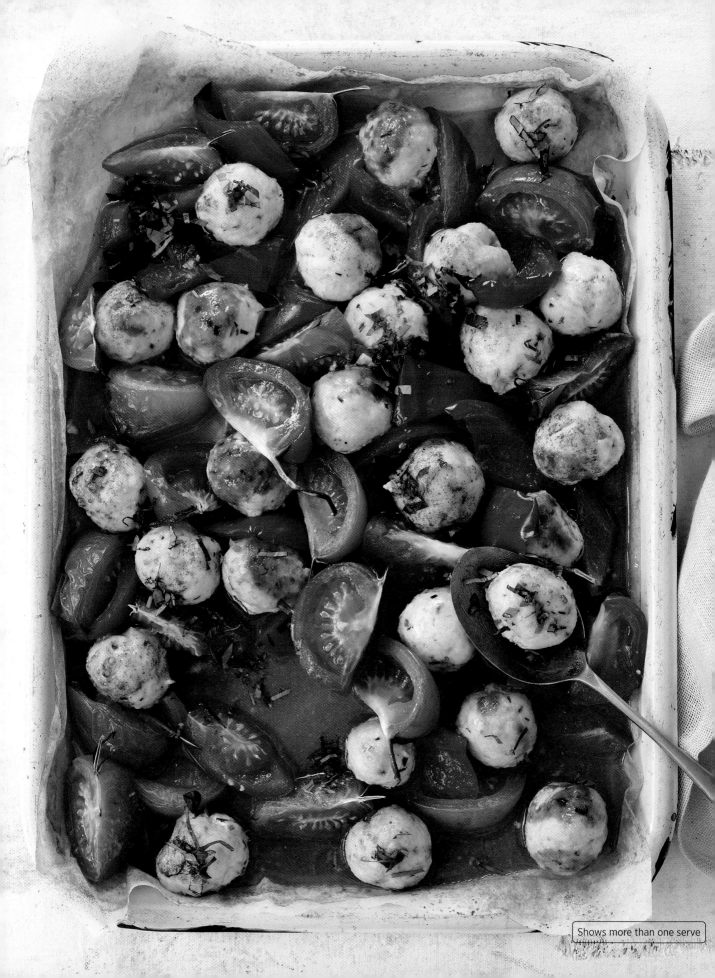

Shows more than one serve

UNITS PER SERVE

Lean meat, fish, poultry, eggs, tofu: **1**

Dairy and dairy alternatives: **1**

Low–moderate carb vegetables: **3**

Healthy fats: **2**

Chicken meatballs in tomato sauce

🍴 **Serves 4**   🕐 **Preparation: 30–35 minutes, plus standing time**
🍲 **Cooking: 20 minutes**   🍳 **Difficulty: Easy**

575 g lean chicken breast fillets, chopped

80 g ground almonds

2 tablespoons chopped chives

2 teaspoons fennel seeds

1 clove garlic, crushed

80 g cheddar, finely grated

1 egg yolk

2 cups (500 ml) salt-reduced chicken stock, heated

1 tablespoon salt-reduced tomato paste

600 g tomatoes, cut into wedges

300 g seeded red capsicum, chopped

HERB DRIZZLE

1 cup basil leaves, finely chopped

¼ cup flat-leaf parsley leaves, finely chopped

1 teaspoon sweet paprika

2 tablespoons red wine vinegar

To make the herb drizzle, whisk all the ingredients together in a small jug. Season to taste with freshly ground black pepper. Set aside until required.

Preheat the oven to 220°C (200°C fan-forced).

Process the chicken in a food processor until minced. Add the almonds, chives, fennel seeds, garlic, cheese and egg yolk and process until the mixture is well combined, smooth and sticky. Season to taste with freshly ground black pepper. Using slightly damp hands, roll walnut-sized portions of mixture into smooth balls. Transfer to a large heavy-based baking dish.

Whisk together the stock and tomato paste until well combined, then pour around the balls in the dish. Add the tomato and capsicum. Roast for 20 minutes or until the meatballs are cooked through and the liquid has reduced by half. Remove and rest for 5 minutes.

Spoon the herb drizzle over the meatballs and sauce and serve.

> **WEEKS 7–12 CARB EXTRAS**
>
> For an extra 8 g carbs per serve, serve with 480 g (120 g per person) steamed green peas.

Note: Store the cooled meatballs in airtight containers in the refrigerator for up to 2 days or freeze for up to 3 months. Thaw in the refrigerator overnight before reheating to serve.

Lean meat, fish, poultry, eggs, tofu: **1.5**
Low–moderate carb vegetables: **4**
Healthy fats: **3**

Spring chicken stew with zesty avocado

8 G CARB PER SERVE

Serves 4   Preparation: 20–25 minutes, plus standing time
Cooking: 15 minutes   Difficulty: Easy

600 g lean chicken tenderloins, halved lengthways
2 cloves garlic, sliced
¼ cup tarragon leaves
3 sprigs lemon thyme
150 g celery, thinly sliced
150 g baby fennel, thinly sliced
300 g zucchini, sliced into rounds
1 litre salt-reduced chicken stock
300 g asparagus, trimmed, halved lengthways, then halved crossways

ZESTY AVOCADO

160 g avocado, chopped
finely grated zest and juice of 2 limes
40 g pine nuts, toasted and chopped
⅓ cup chervil or chopped chives
1 tablespoon lemon thyme leaves

Combine the chicken, garlic, tarragon, lemon thyme, celery, fennel, zucchini and stock in a large deep frying pan over medium heat. Cook, covered and stirring occasionally, for 15 minutes or until the chicken is cooked and the stock has reduced by one-third.

Remove the pan from the heat and stir in the asparagus. Leave to stand, covered, for 5 minutes. Season with freshly ground black pepper.

Meanwhile, to make the zesty avocado, place all the ingredients in a bowl and roughly mash with a fork. Season to taste with freshly ground black pepper.

Serve the chicken stew with the zesty avocado.

WEEKS 7–12 CARB EXTRAS

For an extra 7 g carbs per serve, add 200 g (50 g per person) drained and rinsed tinned cannellini beans to the stew when you add the asparagus.

Note: Store the cooled stew in airtight containers in the refrigerator for up to 2 days or freeze for up to 3 months. Thaw in the refrigerator overnight before reheating to serve.

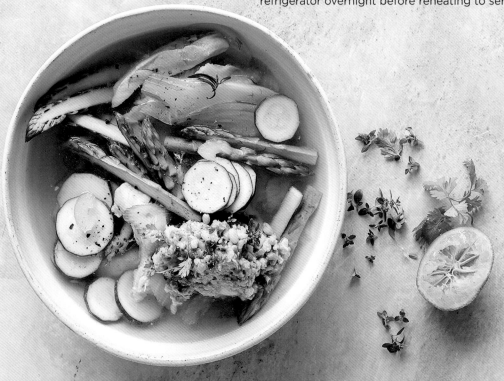

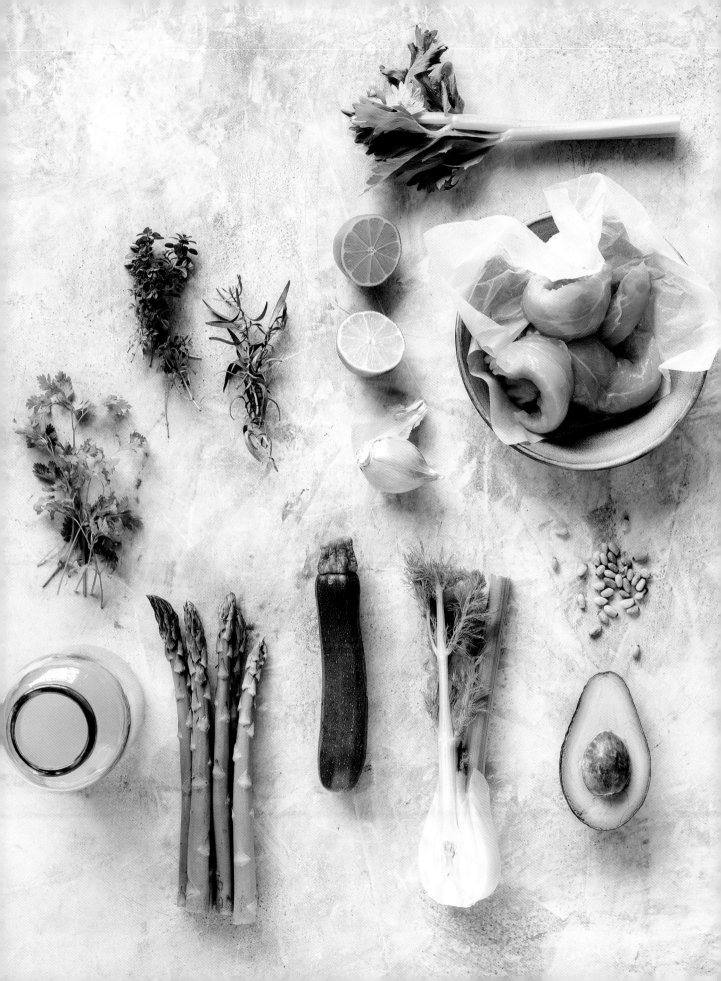

This chapter offers some snacks and sweets
using the carbohydrate extras (such as your fruit
portions), coupled with healthy fat and/or dairy
units, so you can top up your day if needed.
They're also perfect for dinner parties, or if you
just want something a little special in the evening.

SNACKS & SWEETS

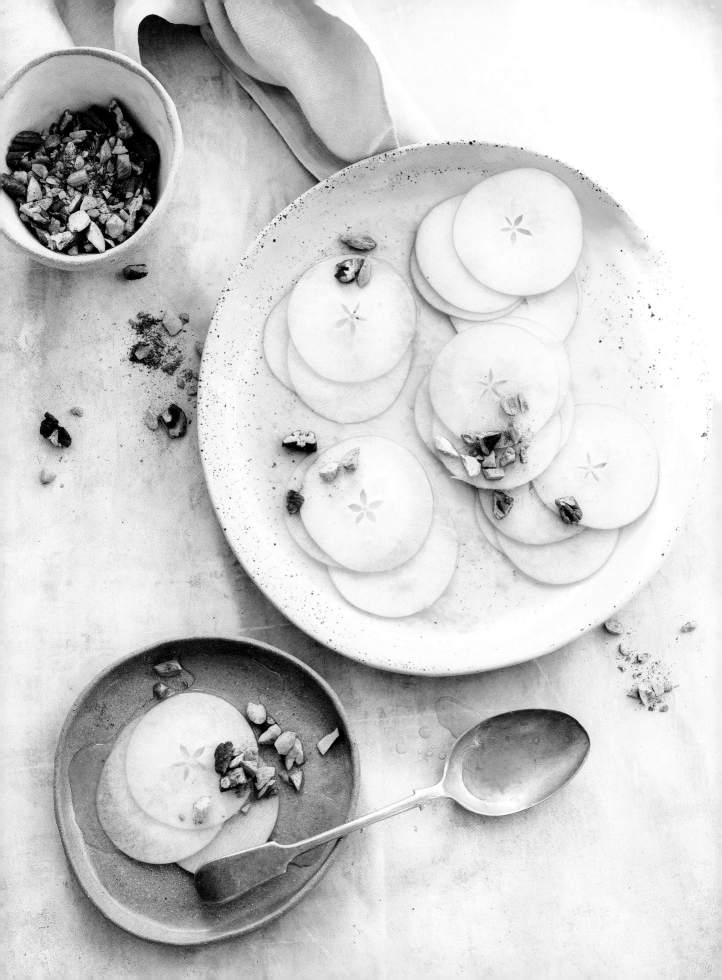

Apple with spiced nut 'crumble'

9 G CARB PER SERVE

🍽 **Serves 4**   🕐 **Preparation: 10–15 minutes**
🍲 **Cooking: 5 minutes**   👩‍🍳 **Difficulty: Easy**

200 g green apple, very thinly sliced into rounds (see note)
finely grated zest and juice of 1 lemon
1 teaspoon pure vanilla extract
40 g blanched almonds
40 g pecans
½ teaspoon mixed spice

Heat a barbecue flat plate to medium.

Combine the apple, lemon zest, juice and vanilla in a bowl, turning so the apple is coated evenly. Arrange the apple slices onto a serving plate.

Mix together the almonds, pecans and mixed spiced. Cook the nut mixture on the flat plate, tossing occasionally, for 2–3 minutes or until evenly golden. Transfer to a board and cool for 2 minutes, then roughly chop.

Sprinkle the chopped nut mixture over the apple slices and serve.

Note: Use a mandoline to very thinly slice the apple into rounds. You will find that the apple seeds will just fall out while slicing.

Raw cinnamon almond 'biscuits'

8 G
CARB
PER
SERVE

🍴 **Serves 8** 🕐 **Preparation: 20–25 minutes, plus standing and chilling time** 🍳 **Cooking: Nil** 👨‍🍳 **Difficulty: Easy**

60 g raw (natural) oats
finely grated zest and juice of
   1 small (200 g) orange
200 g whole natural almonds, toasted
60 g tahini
½ teaspoon ground cinnamon
2 teaspoons pure vanilla extract

Combine the oats, orange juice, almonds, tahini, cinnamon and vanilla in a bowl, then leave to stand for 15 minutes.

Transfer the mixture to a food processor and process until smooth and well combined. Using slightly damp hands, roll 3 teaspoon measures of the mixture into balls and place on a baking tray lined with baking paper (the mixture makes about 22 biscuits). Flatten the balls slightly, then place in the refrigerator for 20 minutes to chill and firm up. Sprinkle with orange zest and serve chilled.

Store in an airtight container in the refrigerator for up to 3 days.

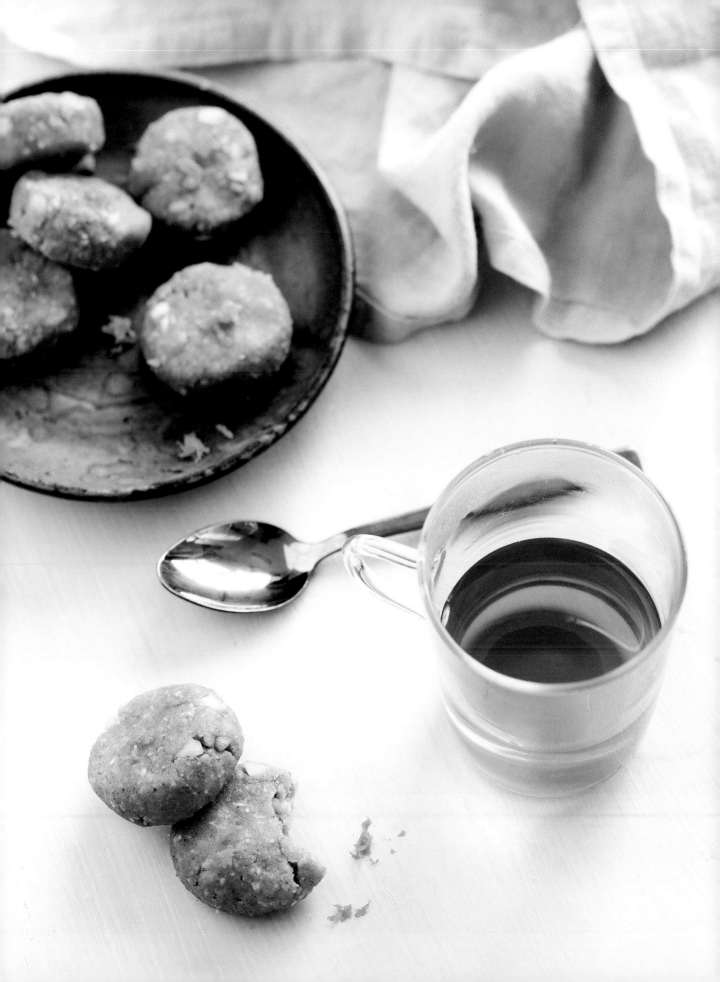

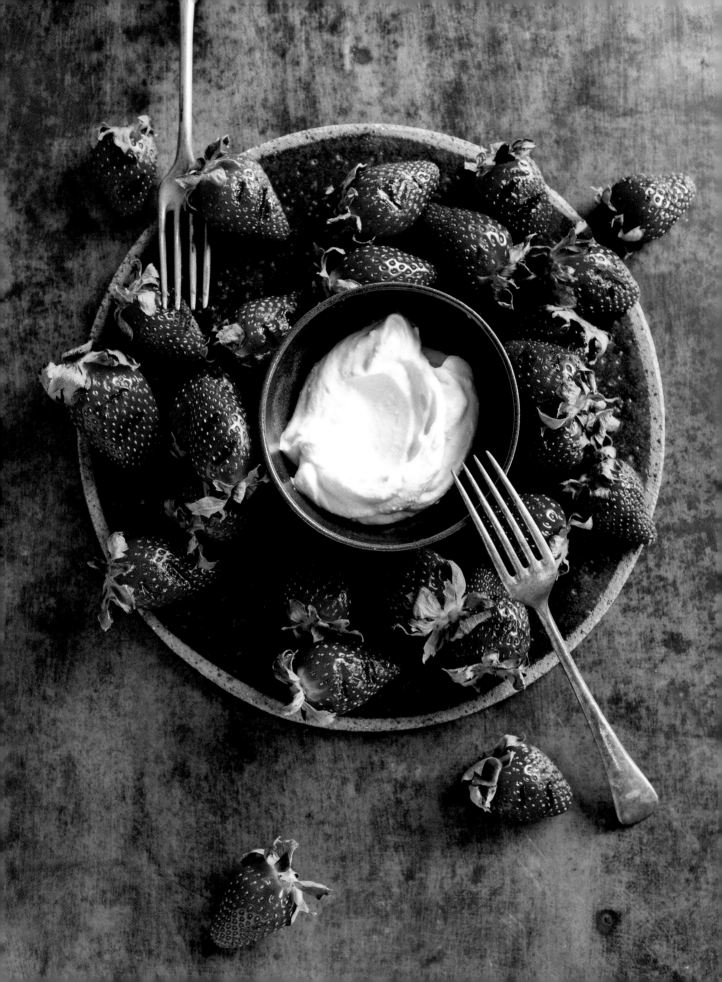

Strawberries with ginger ricotta

🍴 Serves 4   🕐 Preparation: 15–20 minutes
🍲 Cooking: 5 minutes   👨‍🍳 Difficulty: Easy

190 g ricotta
50 g low-fat natural
   Greek-style yoghurt
1 teaspoon pure vanilla extract
1 teaspoon ground ginger
800 g strawberries, halved if large

Heat a barbecue chargrill to high.

Using a hand-held electric mixer, whip the ricotta, yoghurt, vanilla and ginger in a bowl until smooth and creamy. Chill until required.

Cook the strawberries on the chargrill, turning occasionally, for 2 minutes or until golden and heated through.

Divide the strawberries among serving bowls, top with the ginger ricotta and serve.

Note: Strawberries are the only fruit that can also be used as a low–moderate carb vegetable unit. Here they feature as carbohydrate extras.

UNITS PER SERVE
Dairy and dairy alternatives: 1
Carbohydrate extras: 1
Healthy fats: 2

Raspberry and muesli parfaits

13 G CARB PER SERVE

🍴 **Serves 4**   🕐 **Preparation: 10–15 minutes**
〰 **Cooking: 5 minutes**   🍲 **Difficulty: Easy**

30 g untoasted natural muesli
400 g low-fat natural
    Greek-style yoghurt
2 teaspoons pure vanilla extract
¼ teaspoon ground cinnamon
200 g raspberries
80 g toasted mixed nuts (macadamias,
    almonds, pecans)

Heat a barbecue flat plate to medium.

Cook the muesli on the flat plate, tossing occasionally, for 3–4 minutes or until evenly golden. Transfer to a bowl.

Mix together the yoghurt, vanilla and cinnamon in a separate bowl.

Using a fork, crush half the raspberries. Add to the yoghurt mixture and stir until well combined.

Spoon the mixture evenly into serving glasses. Top with the toasted muesli and remaining raspberries and serve.

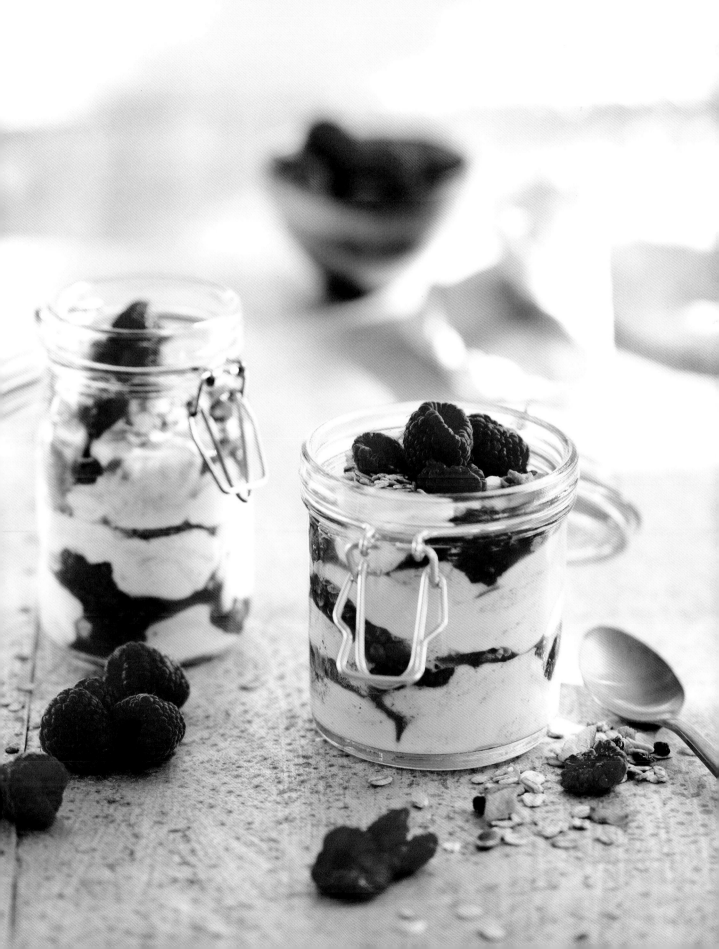

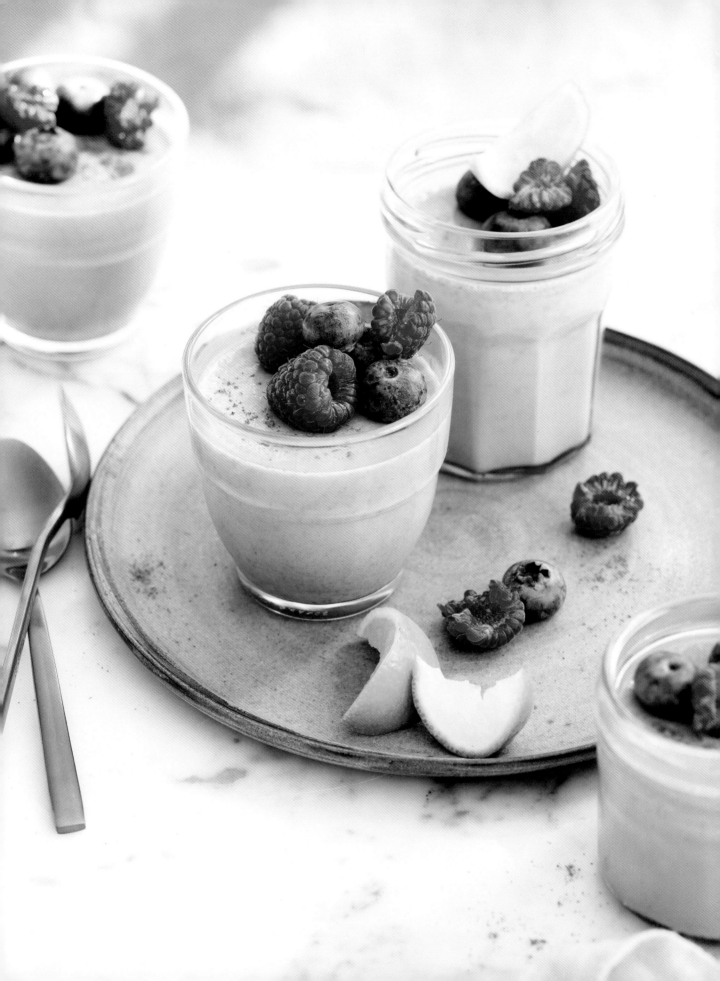

Choc-chilli almond jellies with berries

🍴 **Serves 4**   🕐 **Preparation: 15–20 minutes, plus chilling time**
🌀 **Cooking: 30 seconds**   👍 **Difficulty: Easy**

2 teaspoons cocoa powder
pinch chilli powder, plus extra to serve (optional)
800 ml chilled calcium-enriched almond milk
1 tablespoon powdered gelatine
2 teaspoons pure vanilla extract
200 g raspberries
120 g blueberries
lime wedges, to serve

Combine the cocoa powder, chilli and ½ cup (125 ml) of the almond milk in a microwave-safe jug. Microwave on high for 30 seconds or until hot.

Sprinkle with the gelatine and whisk until the gelatine has dissolved and the mixture is smooth. Whisk in the vanilla and remaining chilled almond milk.

Pour the mixture into four serving glasses and place in the refrigerator for 4 hours or until set.

Arrange the berries over the jellies and serve with lime wedges.

Note: If you don't have a microwave, heat the milk in a small saucepan over low heat without letting it boil.

Dairy and dairy alternatives: **0.5**
Carbohydrate extras: **1**
Healthy fats: **1**

Watermelon, mint and pistachio salad

7 G
CARB
PER
SERVE

🍴 **Serves 4**   🕐 **Preparation: 10–15 minutes, plus chilling time**
🍲 **Cooking: Nil**   👨‍🍳 **Difficulty: Easy**

400 g peeled seedless watermelon,
　cut into small triangles
40 g feta, crumbled
40 g unsalted shelled pistachios,
　toasted, finely chopped
2 teaspoons rosewater
½ cup mint leaves
½ cup tarragon leaves

Gently combine all the ingredients in a serving bowl and chill for 15 minutes. Serve.

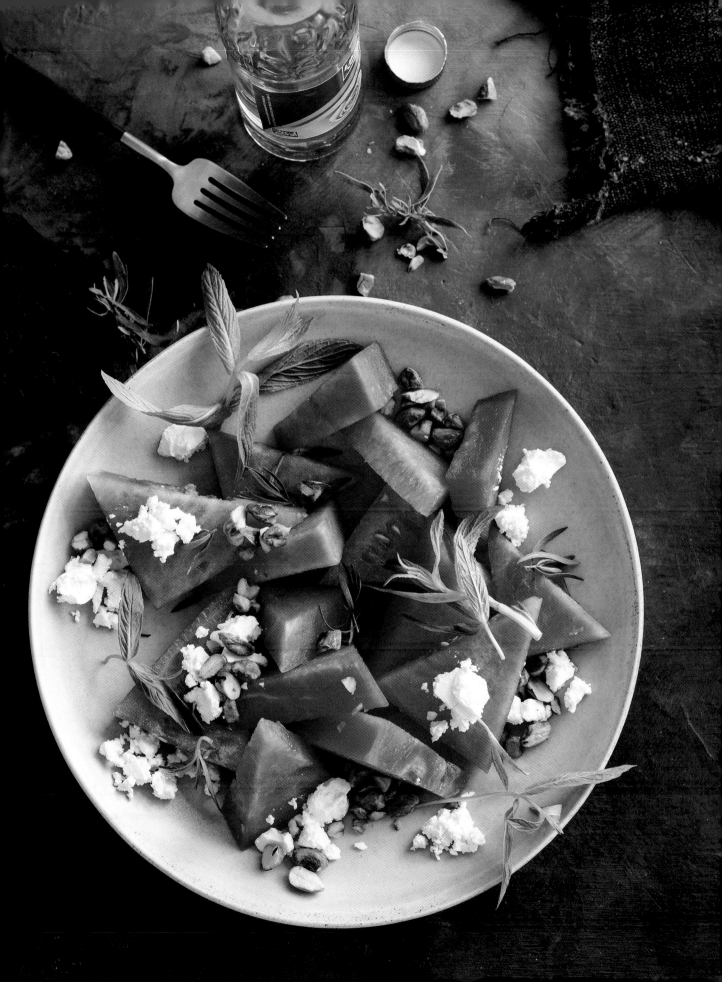

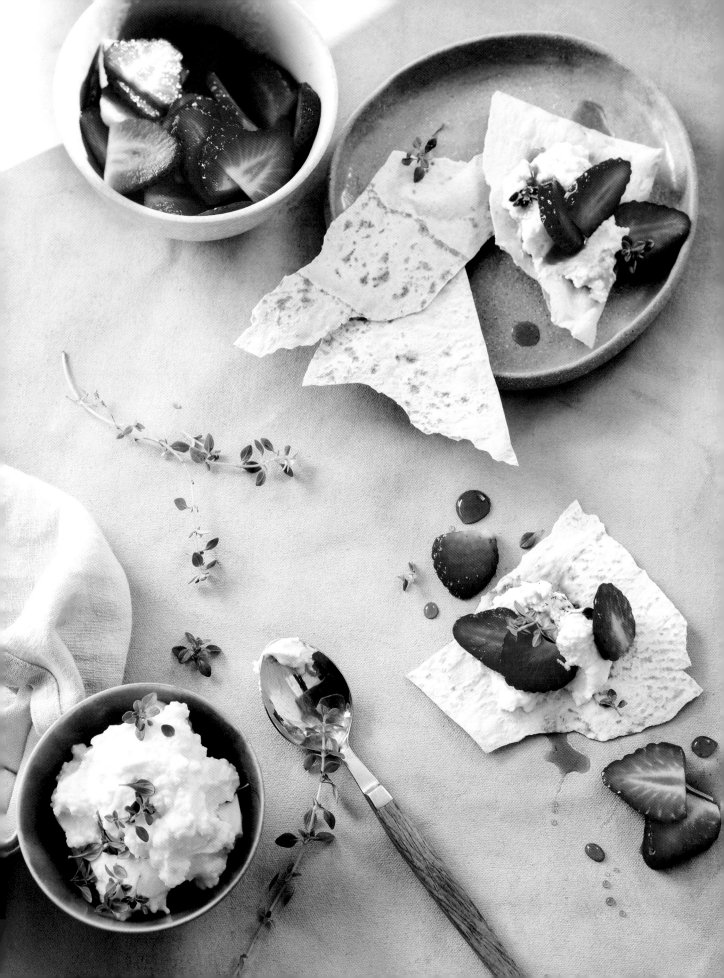

Lemon thyme ricotta with vanilla strawberries

🍴 **Serves 4**   🕐 **Preparation: 20–25 minutes, plus standing and cooling time**   🍳 **Cooking: 5 minutes**   👩‍🍳 **Difficulty: Easy**

2 multigrain mountain breads
220 g ricotta
2 teaspoons pure vanilla extract
2 teaspoons lemon thyme leaves

VANILLA STRAWBERRIES
200 g strawberries, hulled and sliced
2 tablespoons red wine vinegar
2 teaspoons pure vanilla extract

Preheat the oven to 180°C (160°C fan-forced).

Bake the mountain bread directly on the oven rack for 3–5 minutes or until crisp and light golden. Transfer to a board and cool, then break into shards for serving.

Meanwhile, to make the vanilla strawberries, combine all the ingredients in a bowl. Leave to macerate for 15 minutes, stirring occasionally.

Mix together the ricotta, vanilla and lemon thyme in a bowl, then spread over the mountain bread shards. Spoon over the vanilla strawberries and their juices and serve immediately.

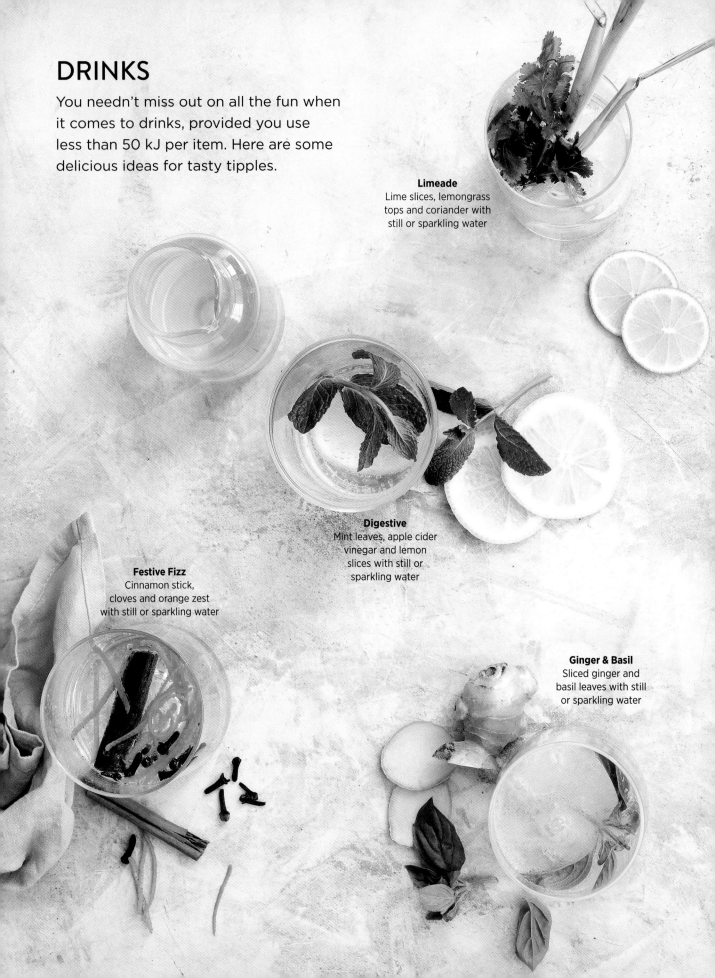

DRINKS

You needn't miss out on all the fun when it comes to drinks, provided you use less than 50 kJ per item. Here are some delicious ideas for tasty tipples.

Limeade
Lime slices, lemongrass tops and coriander with still or sparkling water

Digestive
Mint leaves, apple cider vinegar and lemon slices with still or sparkling water

Festive Fizz
Cinnamon stick, cloves and orange zest with still or sparkling water

Ginger & Basil
Sliced ginger and basil leaves with still or sparkling water

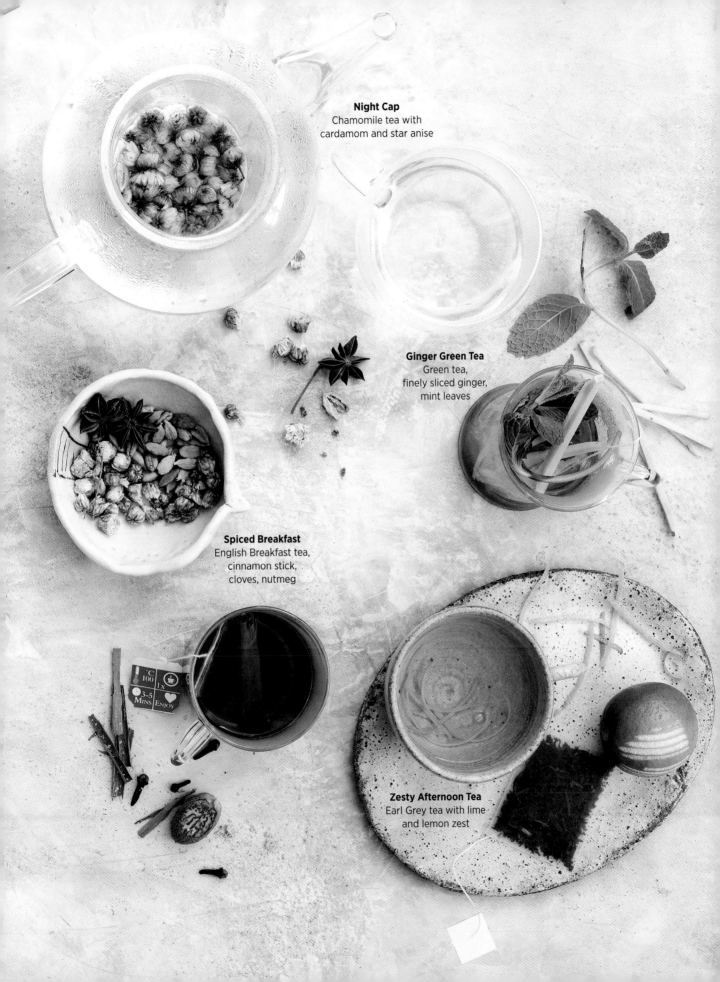

Night Cap
Chamomile tea with
cardamom and star anise

Ginger Green Tea
Green tea,
finely sliced ginger,
mint leaves

Spiced Breakfast
English Breakfast tea,
cinnamon stick,
cloves, nutmeg

Zesty Afternoon Tea
Earl Grey tea with lime
and lemon zest

PART 3

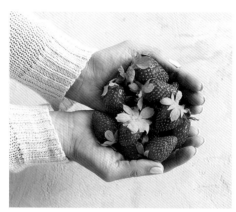

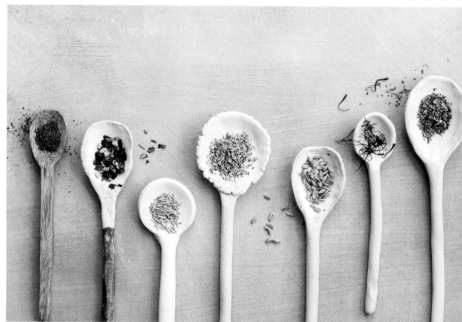

Aim for at least three aerobic exercise sessions per week.

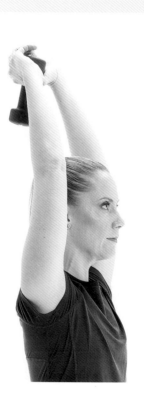

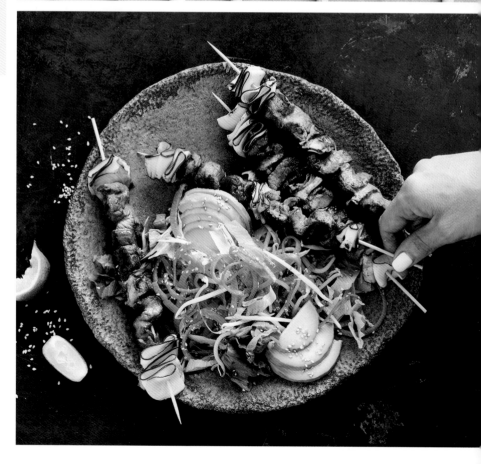

The CSIRO Exercise Plan

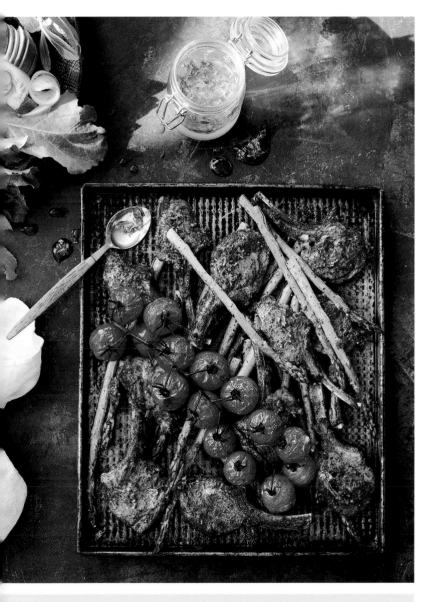

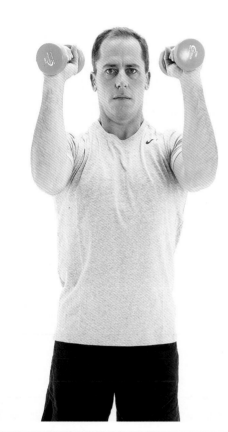

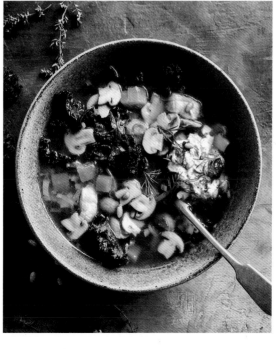

Try to reduce the time spent sitting throughout the day, and increase the amount of incidental physical activity you do.

BENEFITS OF EXERCISING

Watching your diet is vital to managing your weight and improving your health; however, regular physical activity plays an equally important role and is a core component of a comprehensive lifestyle program.

Exercise boosts health and wellbeing

A high level of physical activity is one of the best predictors of maintaining weight loss over the long term. Evidence consistently shows that increased physical activity is also associated with numerous health benefits, including:

- improved blood glucose control
- reduced risk of cardiovascular disease, type 2 diabetes and premature death
- lower blood pressure and blood fat levels
- reduced rates of some forms of cancer, depression and osteoporosis.

Evidence also shows that these health benefits are achieved regardless of whether or not you lose weight.

Therefore, the greatest benefits of the CSIRO Low-carb Diet are achieved by also participating in regular exercise and enjoying a physically active lifestyle.

> Before starting a new exercise program, it is a good idea to consult your healthcare team to check it is safe for you to start exercising, particularly if you have a pre-existing condition like diabetes, or any physical limitations. An accredited exercise physiologist will be able to help tailor an exercise program to meet your individual needs and abilities.

The main types of exercise

An exercise program that provides the best overall mix of health benefits will include the following three types of exercise.

1. Aerobic exercise

Also known as endurance exercise or cardiorespiratory fitness training (cardio), aerobic exercise involves sustained activities that use large muscle groups in a rhythmic manner, such as walking, swimming and cycling. This type of exercise helps to stabilise blood glucose and improves aerobic fitness, which reduces the risk of premature death.

2. Resistance training

Also known as strength training, this form of training consists of shorter, more intense activities that promote increases in muscle mass, strength, speed and power. These activities typically involve overloading the muscles with some kind of weight, such as your body weight or a dumbbell.

This type of exercise increases muscle mass (or slows age-related muscle mass loss), which enhances strength and metabolism, helps to stabilise blood glucose and increases bone strength. Maintaining a higher metabolic rate will help you to burn more energy at rest, making it easier to maintain a healthier body weight.

3. Flexibility training

Also commonly referred to as stretching, flexibility training involves stretching or repeatedly moving a joint through its complete range of motion. This type of exercise can prevent the loss of joint range of motion, which makes the other types of exercise easier to perform, and improves general quality of life.

Your weekly exercise program

Rating of perceived exertion of exercise session	
0	Rest
1	Very, very easy
2	Easy
3	Moderate
4	Somewhat hard
5	Hard
6	–
7	Very hard
8	–
9	–
10	Maximum

Source: C Foster et al., 'A new approach to monitoring exercise training', *Journal of Strength and Conditioning Research*, 2001, vol. 15, no. 1, pp. 109–15.

Your suggested exercise plan for the CSIRO Low-carb Diet incorporates all three forms of exercise above, set out as follows.

1. Aerobic exercise component

Aim for at least three aerobic exercise sessions per week, of moderate or higher (vigorous) intensity.

This could include easier activities such as brisk walking to begin with, as well as other activities like jogging, cycling, rowing, aerobics, swimming and so on.

If you are only starting, it is best to begin with short sessions of about 30 minutes and build up progressively over several weeks, to sessions of 55–60 minutes in duration.

Your goal should be to achieve at least 150 minutes of moderate-intensity aerobic exercise each week, or 75 minutes of vigorous-intensity aerobic exercise per week.

CHECK YOUR EXERCISE INTENSITY

For both the aerobic exercise and resistance training sessions, you can keep track of the relative intensity of your workout (i.e. the overall difficulty of the entire exercise session) using a number from the table opposite. A moderate-intensity workout, which you should be aiming for as a minimum, corresponds to a rating of 3.

2. Resistance training component

Aim for at least two resistance training sessions per week, on non-consecutive days. These sessions should consist of 8–10 exercises, including:

- 3–4 upper-body exercises
- 3–4 lower-body exercises
- 2 core exercises.

Over the next pages we outline some resistance exercises you can use in your routine to provide greater variety and help you stay motivated, as well as some more advanced options to ensure you continue to improve your strength and fitness and benefit fully from the program. (You will also find a whole series of suitable exercises in Part 4 of our first book, *The CSIRO Low-carb Diet*.)

When performing your resistance exercises, a good pace to conduct them at is a tempo of 2:1:2 seconds (effort:hold:release). For example, for the Floor Chest Press on page 232, this would mean taking 2 seconds to lower the dumbbell, holding the dumbbell at the bottom for 1 second, then taking 2 seconds to return the dumbbell to the starting position.

Aim to perform two to three sets of each exercise in your workout, allowing yourself a 1–2 minute rest between sets.

REMEMBER YOUR BREATHING

While doing your resistance exercises, remember not to hold your breath. Aim to **breathe out** during the effort phase (i.e. when the muscle is shortening under tension, such as when you are lifting a dumbbell), and **breathe in** during the release phase, when the muscle is lengthened under tension (such as when you are lowering the dumbbell).

3. Warm-up and cool-down

Start and end each exercise session with a 5–10 minute warm-up of gentle aerobic activities to prepare your body for exercise, as well as a 5–10 minute cool-down, incorporating a range of flexibility exercises that stretch the major muscle groups (see book 1 for a full range of these).

PROGRESSIVE OVERLOAD

As you become fitter and stronger, and the activities become easier to perform, it is important to gradually increase the difficulty of the activity, to continue to improve and fully benefit from the exercise program.

Just keep moving

Research shows that, independent of the amount of physical activity you do, the amount of time you spend being inactive can be a separate risk factor for developing diabetes and heart disease.

For your health, then, it is important to take every opportunity to be active, and reduce the amount of time you spend being sedentary each day.

As well as participating in a regular structured exercise program, try to reduce the time spent sitting or lying down throughout the day, and increase the amount of incidental physical activity you do.

Some simple ways to incorporate extra activity into your day is by walking upstairs instead of taking the lift, standing rather than sitting when talking on the phone, taking a short walk during your coffee break, and standing up and moving around during television ad breaks.

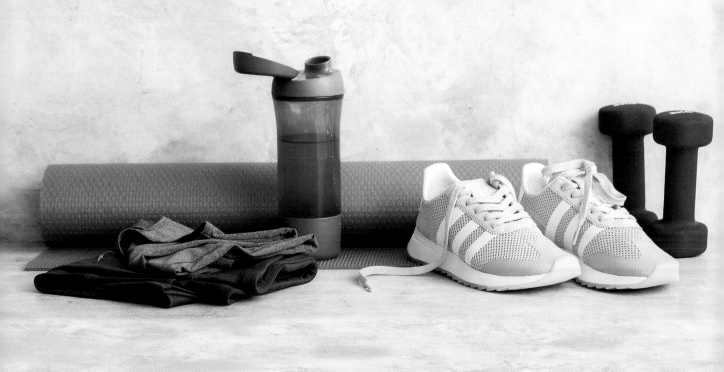

UPPER BODY

1.
Floor chest press

For Chest/triceps **Weight** Dumbbells

Start position Lie down on the floor, on your back, with your knees bent at around 90 degrees and feet flat on the floor. Hold a dumbbell in each hand, with your elbows extended straight out in front of your chest, and palms facing each other. The dumbbells should be approximately chest-width apart.

1. Breathe in and bend your elbows to slowly lower the weights, without rotating your hands, until your upper arm contacts the floor. Your elbows should finish alongside your body, with your upper arms parallel to your body.

2. Breathe out and lift, and extend your elbows, pushing the dumbbells straight up to the start position.

Tip You can begin by resting the dumbbells on your thighs, and do a gentle knee raise to help lift the dumbbells one at a time to the start position.

Variations To concentrate on your chest muscles, perform the exercise starting with your palms facing forward and lower the weights with your elbows pointing outwards (finishing with your upper arms perpendicular to your body).

2.
Shoulder press

For Shoulder (deltoid) **Weight** Dumbbells

Start position Holding a dumbbell in each hand, stand upright with your upper arms perpendicular to the side of your body, your elbows bent at 90 degrees, your lower arms perpendicular to the floor, and your palms facing forward.

1. Breathe out and, keeping your torso still, extend and raise both elbows, lifting the dumbbells above head height.

2. Breathe in and lower the dumbbells back down slowly to the start position.

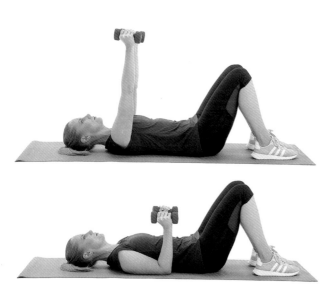
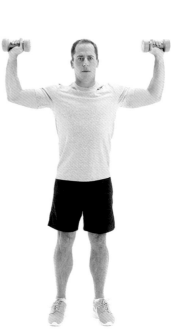
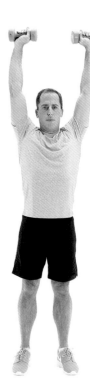

3.
Triceps press

For Triceps **Weight** Dumbbell

Start position Stand upright, holding a single dumbbell with both hands. The dumbbell should be held cupped by its head so your palms are facing up. Raise the dumbbell to lift it over your head, with both arms fully extended and perpendicular to the floor.

1. Breathe in and, while keeping your upper arms stationary, bend the elbows to slowly lower the dumbbell behind your head until your elbows are fully flexed.

2. Breathe out and extend your elbows to lift the weight back to the start position.

4.
Shoulder raise

For Shoulder (deltoid) **Weight** Dumbbells

Start position Stand upright, with a dumbbell in each hand, and your arms slightly out from the side of your body. Your elbows should be close to your torso, and your palms should be facing forward.

1. Breathe out and, keeping your torso still, lift both arms outwards and upwards without bending your elbows. Continue to lift up until your arms are parallel to the floor.

2. Breathe in and slowly lower the dumbbells back down to the start position.

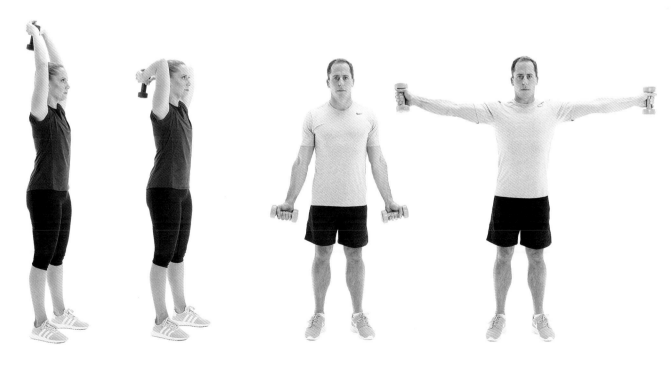

UPPER BODY

5.

Shrugs

For Upper back (trapezius) **Weight** Dumbbells

Start position Stand upright with your arms by your side, and a dumbbell in each hand. Your elbows should be close to your torso, and your palms should be facing your thighs.

1. Breathe out and slowly elevate your shoulders as high as possible, while keeping your arms by your side.

2. Breathe in and slowly lower your shoulders back to the start position.

6.

Standing pec fly

For Chest/shoulders **Weight** Dumbbells

Start position Holding a dumbbell in each hand, stand upright with your upper arms perpendicular to the side of your body, your elbows bent at 90 degrees, your lower arms perpendicular to the floor, and your palms facing forward.

1. Breathe out and bring your arms and elbows inwards in front of your chest, while maintaining the 90-degree elbow bend and keeping your upper arms perpendicular to the floor.

2. Breathe in and slowly return to the start position.

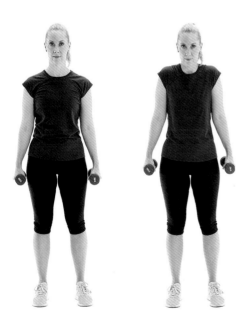
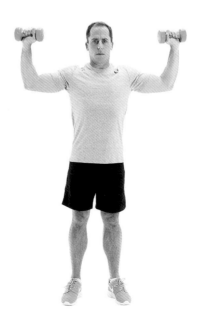
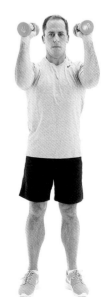

LOWER BODY

7.

Rear deltoid fly

For Shoulder (deltoid) **Weight** Dumbbells

Start position Stand upright with your knees bent slightly. Bend forward at the waist so you are leaning over your feet. Hold a dumbbell in each hand (palms facing each other), with your arms hanging down in front of you with a slight elbow bend. Keep your head up and facing slightly forward.

1. Breathe out and, keeping your torso stationary and your arms extended, lift both dumbbells outwards and upwards until your arms are parallel to the floor.

2. Breathe in and slowly lower the dumbbells back to the start position.

8.

Deadlift

For Hamstrings **Weight** Dumbbells

Start position Stand upright with your arms pointing down in front of you, and a dumbbell in each hand. Your palms should be facing the front of your thighs, and your weight should be on your heels.

1. Breathe in and, keeping your body weight on your heels, and your arms down, bend at the hips to push your bottom backwards as far as possible, keeping your torso and stomach tight. Your knees should bend just a little, and you should keep your chest up and your back arched inwards.

2. Breathe out and slowly bring the hips forward to return to the start position.

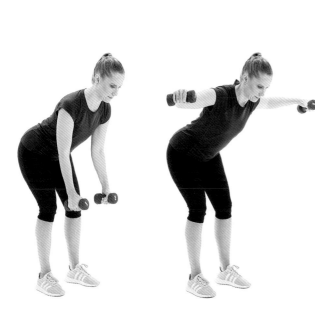
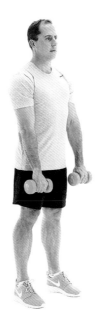
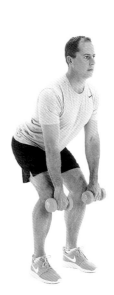

LOWER BODY

9.
Side lunge

For Quads **Weight** Body weight/dumbbell

Start position Stand upright with your feet shoulder-width apart.

1. Breathe in and, while maintaining an upright posture, take a moderate-sized, low step sideways with your right foot, pointing your toes slightly outward. Shift your body weight onto your right heel and bend your right knee to slowly squat down as low as you are able. Keep your chest up high and your left knee extended to the side.

2. Breathe out and push back up from your right foot, bringing yourself back to the start position.

3. Repeat the movement with the left foot stepping sideways. A complete left- and right-side sequence equals 1 repetition.

Bodyweight version Clasp your hands together in front of your chest, with your elbows bent.

Dumbbell (advanced) version Hold a dumbbell between your hands (palms facing each other) in front of your chest, with your elbows bent.

10.
Goblet squat

For Quads **Weight** Body weight/dumbbell

Start position Stand upright with your feet shoulder-width apart.

1. Breathe in and flex your knees and hips so you are sitting back, keeping your weight on your heels, and your knees behind the front of your toes. Keep your head and chest up high, and your bottom out during the movement. Squat down as low as you are able, or until your knees are at a 90-degree angle.

2. Breathe out and reverse the motion, coming back to the start position.

Bodyweight version Clasp your hands together in front of your chest, with your elbows bent.

Dumbbell (advanced) version Hold a dumbbell between your hands (palms facing each other) in front of your chest, with your elbows bent.

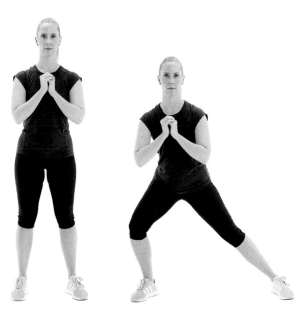

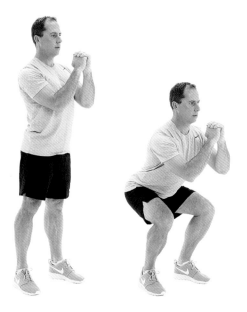

CORE & LOWER BODY

CORE

11.

Woodchop

For Abdominals, quads & glutes **Weight** Dumbbell

Start position Stand with your feet shoulder-width apart. Clasp a single dumbbell with both hands. Raise the dumbbell above head height and out to the right-hand side of your body, with your arms fully extended.

1. Breathe in and, keeping your arms straight, bring the dumbbell down diagonally across your body, keeping your head and chest up, and bending your hips and knees to squat down as you go. Finish with the dumbbell to the side of your left leg at knee height.

2. Breathe out and reverse the movement to finish back at the start position. Repeat for the desired number of repetitions.

3. After one full set, repeat on the other side, starting with the dumbbell up and to the left.

12.

Side plank/hip raise

For Abdominals **Weight** Body weight

Start position Lie on your left side, with your right foot stacked on top of your left foot. Use your right hand to assist in propping your body up on your left elbow and forearm. Your elbow should be located directly below your shoulder. Place your right hand on your hip and raise your hips so your body forms a straight line from your ankles to your shoulders.

1. Breathing continuously, keep your body straight and hold this position for at least 10 seconds.

2. Repeat the movement lying on your right-hand side.

Easier variation Bend your knees 90 degrees and use your knee as the pivot point.

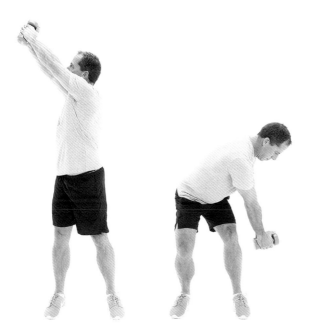

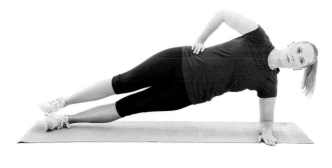

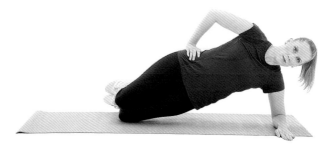

CORE

13.
Ab twist

For Abdominals **Weight** Body weight/dumbbell

Start position Lie down on the floor, on your back, with your knees bent at 90 degrees. Lift your feet about 10 cm off the ground and sit up so your torso and thighs are at 90 degrees. Clasp your hands together in front of you, with your arms straight.

1. Breathing constantly and keeping your legs stationary, twist your torso to the right, keeping your arms parallel to the ground.

2. Now twist your torso around to the left, keeping your arms parallel to the ground. A complete right- and left-side sequence equals 1 repetition.

Easier variation Pin your feet under something heavy, or have a partner hold them down.

Advanced version Hold a dumbbell for added resistance.

14.
Jack-knife sit-up

For Abdominals **Weight** Body weight

Start position Lie down on the floor on your back, with your legs straight and your arms extended behind your head.

1. Breathe out and bend at the waist to bring your legs up, while simultaneously bringing your arms over your head and reaching up towards your feet, lifting your upper torso as you go. Keep your arms and legs straight throughout the movement.

2. Breathe in and slowly return back to the start position.

Advanced version Hold a dumbbell for added resistance.

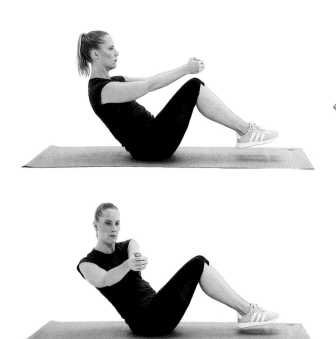

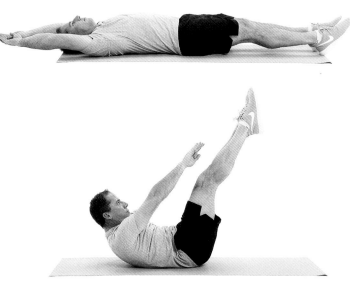

15.

Bent-knee hip raise

For Abdominals/hamstrings **Weight** Body weight

Start position Lie down on the floor on your back, with your knees bent at 90 degrees and your arms by your sides, palms facing down.

1. Breathe out and, while maintaining the bend in your knees, bring your legs up and over your chest, lifting your hips up off the floor as you go.

2. Breathe in and slowly return to the start position.

Advanced version Keep your legs straight.

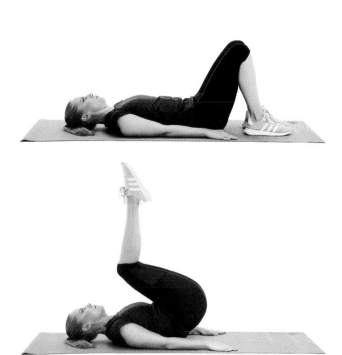

APPENDIX A:
CALCULATING HEALTH MEASURES

What is your BMI?

If you prefer to use an online tool to calculate your BMI, visit:
healthyweight.health.gov.au/wps/portal/Home/helping-hand/bmi

Are you at risk of cardiovascular disease?

To complete the online Australian Absolute Cardiovascular disease risk questionnaire, visit: cvdcheck.org.au. You'll need your latest blood pressure and blood cholesterol readings.

Do you have type 2 diabetes?

The Australian type 2 diabetes risk assessment tool (AusDRISK) was created by the Baker IDI Heart and Diabetes Institute to help health practitioners and the general public determine their risk of developing the condition. Check your risk now by answering the questions opposite, or complete the online assessment at: diabetesaustralia.com.au/are-you-at-risk-type-2

Calculating your basal metabolic rate

To determine your BMR online, go to the Australian Government's calculator at: eatforhealth.gov.au/node/add/calculator-energy

Diabetes risk assessment

1. What is your age group?

Under 35	0 points
35–44	2 points
45–54	4 points
55–64	6 points
65 or over	8 points

2. What is your gender?

Female	0 points
Male	3 points

3. What are your ethnicity and your country of birth?

Are you of Aboriginal, Torres Strait Islander, Pacific Islander or Maori descent?

No	0 points
Yes	2 points

Where were you born?

Australia	0 points
Asia	2 points
Indian subcontinent	2 points
Middle East	2 points
North Africa	2 points
Southern Europe	2 points
Other	0 points

4. Have either of your parents, or any of your brothers or sisters, been diagnosed with diabetes (type 1 or type 2)?

No	0 points
Yes	3 points

5. Have you ever been found to have high blood glucose (sugar) in a health examination, during an illness or during pregnancy?

No	0 points
Yes	6 points

6. Are you currently taking medication for high blood pressure?

No	0 points
Yes	2 points

7. Do you currently smoke cigarettes or any other tobacco products on a daily basis?

No	0 points
Yes	2 points

8. How often do you eat vegetables or fruit?

Every day	0 points
Not every day	1 point

9. On average, would you say you do at least 2.5 hours of physical activity per week (for example, 30 minutes a day on five or more days a week)?

Yes	0 points
No	2 points

10. What is your waist measurement taken below the ribs (usually at the level of the navel, and while standing)?

For those of Asian or Aboriginal or Torres Strait Islander descent

Men	Women	
Less than 90 cm	Less than 80 cm	0 points
90–100 cm	80–90 cm	4 points
More than 100 cm	More than 90 cm	7 points

For all others

Men	Women	
Less than 102 cm	Less than 88 cm	0 points
102–110 cm	88–100 cm	4 points
More than 110 cm	More than 100 cm	7 points

Your risk of developing type 2 diabetes within 5 years

Check your total score against the three point ranges below. Note that if you're less than 25 years old, the overall score may overestimate your risk of diabetes.

5 or less: Low risk

Approximately one person in every 100 with a score in this range will develop diabetes.

6–11: Intermediate risk

Approximately one person in every 50 with a score in the range of 6–8 will develop diabetes. Approximately one person in every 30 with a score in the range of 9–11 will develop diabetes. Discuss your score with your GP and consider lifestyle changes to reduce your risk.

12 or more: High risk

Approximately one person in every 14 with a score in the range of 12–15 will develop diabetes. Approximately one person in every seven with a score in the range of 16–19 will develop diabetes. Approximately one person in every three with a score in the range of 20 and above will develop diabetes. You may have undiagnosed diabetes. See your GP as soon as possible for a fasting glucose test.

APPENDIX B:
TRAINING DIARY TEMPLATES

Resistance exercises

Week:			Date: ___ /___ /___		
Day: Monday Tuesday Wednesday Thursday Friday Saturday Sunday					
Session rating of perceived exertion (see page 229):					
General comments:					
Region	Exercise name	Body weight or dumbbell (kg)	Repetitions		
			Set 1	Set 2	Set 3
Upper body	**e.g. push-up**	**body weight**	**12**	**9**	**8**
Core					
Lower body					

Aerobic exercises

Week	Day (circle)	Date	Activity	Duration (mins)	Session rating of perceived exertion (see page 229)	General comments
1	M Tu W Th F Sa Su	__ /__ /__	**e.g. walking**	**35**	**3**	
	M Tu W Th F Sa Su	__ /__ /__				
	M Tu W Th F Sa Su	__ /__ /__				
	M Tu W Th F Sa Su	__ /__ /__				
	M Tu W Th F Sa Su	__ /__ /__				
2	M Tu W Th F Sa Su	__ /__ /__				
	M Tu W Th F Sa Su	__ /__ /__				
	M Tu W Th F Sa Su	__ /__ /__				
	M Tu W Th F Sa Su	__ /__ /__				
	M Tu W Th F Sa Su	__ /__ /__				
	M Tu W Th F Sa Su	__ /__ /__				
3	M Tu W Th F Sa Su	__ /__ /__				
	M Tu W Th F Sa Su	__ /__ /__				
	M Tu W Th F Sa Su	__ /__ /__				
	M Tu W Th F Sa Su	__ /__ /__				
	M Tu W Th F Sa Su	__ /__ /__				
	M Tu W Th F Sa Su	__ /__ /__				

Acknowledgements

First, we'd like to thank our scientific co-investigators and collaborators for their contributions to our scientific ideas, their guidance and their commitment to this important research topic: Dr Jeannie Tay, CSIRO and Agency for Science Technology and Research (A*Star), Singapore; Professor Jon Buckley, University of South Australia; Professor Gary Wittert, University of Adelaide; Associate Professor William Yancy Jr, Duke University, United States; Professor Carlene Wilson, Flinders University, South Australia; Dr Vanessa Danthiir, CSIRO; Dr Ian Zajac, CSIRO; and Professor Peter Clifton, University of South Australia.

We thank the following individuals of the Clinical Research Team at CSIRO Health and Biosecurity, Adelaide, South Australia, for their tireless work in conducting the clinical research activities that underpin the contents of this book: Anne McGuffin, Julia Weaver, and Vanessa Courage for coordinating the research trials; Janna Lutze, Dr Paul Foster, Xenia Cleantheous, Gemma Williams, Hannah Gilbert and Fiona Barr for assisting in designing and implementing the dietary interventions; Lindy Lawson, Theresa McKinnon, Rosemary McArthur and Heather Webb for nursing expertise and clinical patient management; Vanessa Russell, Cathryn Pape, Candita Dang, Andre Nikolic and Sylvia Usher for performing biochemical assays and for other laboratory expertise; Julie Syrette and Kathryn Bastiaans for data management; Kylie Lange and Mary Barnes for assisting with statistical analyses; Andreas Kahl for communications; and our external fitness partners and health coaches for implementing the exercise interventions, including Luke Johnston and Annie Hastwell of Fit for Success, South Australia; Kelly French, Jason Delfos, Kristi Lacey-Powell, Marilyn Woods, John Perrin, Simon Pane and Annette Beckette of South Australian Aquatic and Leisure Centre; and Angie Mondello and Josh Gniadek of Boot Camp Plus, South Australia.

Thanks to the editorial and publishing team at Pan Macmillan Australia: Ingrid Ohlsson, who supported the writing of this book with great enthusiasm and encouragement; Virginia Birch, Megan Pigott, Naomi Van Groll and Sally Devenish for their tireless work and support through the editorial and publication process. Thanks also to designer Susanne Geppert, editor Katri Hilden, recipe developer and home economist Tracey Pattison, recipe editor Rachel Carter, photographer Jeremy Simons, stylist Michelle Noerianto, exercise models Annie Smith and Bjorn Shakespeare, and Coco Stallman, Tammi Kwok and Pam Dunne.

Finally, and most importantly, we'd like to thank the research volunteers for their participation in our research trials. It's only through their contributions that our research and these significant advancements in clinical practices for weight and diabetes management have been made possible.

A complete bibliography can be found in *The CSIRO Low-carb Diet*.

Index

First published 2018 in Macmillan
by Pan Macmillan Australia Pty Limited
1 Market Street, Sydney, New South Wales
Australia 2000

A CIP catalogue record for this book is available from the National Library of Australia: http://catalogue.nla.gov.au

Original design concept by Daniel New / Oetomo New
Design by Susanne Geppert
Photography by Jeremy Simons
Prop and food styling by Michelle Noerianto
Recipe development by Tracey Pattison
Editing by Katri Hilden and Rachel Carter
Colour + reproduction by Splitting Image Colour Studio
Printed in China by 1010 Printing International Limited